ELSEVIER

1600 John F. Kennedy Boulevard • Suite 1800 • Philadelphia, Pennsylvania, 19103-2899
http://www.theclinics.com

RHEUMATIC DISEASE CLINICS OF NORTH AMERICA Volume 46, Number 4
November 2020 ISSN 0889-857X, ISBN 13: 978-0-323-79601-9

Editor: Lauren Boyle
Developmental Editor: Casey Potter

Rheumatic Disease Clinics of North America (ISSN 0889-857X) is published quarterly by Elsevier Inc., 360 Park
Avenue South, New York, NY 10010-1710. Months of issue are February, May, August, and November. Business
and editorial offices: 1600 John F. Kennedy Boulevard, Suite 1800, Philadelphia, PA 19103-2899. Periodicals
postage paid at New York, NY and additional mailing offices. Subscription prices are USD 362.00 per year for
US individuals, USD 777.00 per year for US institutions, USD 100.00 per year for US students and residents,
USD 427.00 per year for Canadian individuals, USD 971.00 per year for Canadian institutions, USD 100.00 per
year for Canadian students/residents, USD 465.00 per year for international individuals, USD 971.00 per year
for international institutions, and USD 230.00 per year for foreign students/residents. To receive student/resident
rate, orders must be accompanied by name of affiliated institution, date of term, and the *signature* of program/
residency coordinator on institution letterhead. Orders will be billed at individual rate until proof of status received. Foreign air speed delivery is included in all *Clinics* subscription prices. All prices are subject to change
without notice. **POSTMASTER:** Send address changes to *Rheumatic Disease Clinics of North America,* Elsevier
Health Sciences Division, Subscription Customer Service, 3251 Riverport Lane, Maryland Heights, MO 63043.
**Customer Service: 1-800-654-2452 (US and Canada). From outside of the US and Canada: 314-447-
8871. Fax: 314-447-8029. For print support, e-mail: JournalsCustomerService-usa@elsevier.com. For online support, e-mail: JournalsOnlineSupport-usa@elsevier.com.**

Reprints. For copies of 100 or more of articles in this publication, please contact the Commercial Reprints
Department, Elsevier Inc., 360 Park Avenue South, New York, New York, 10010-1710; Tel.: +1-212-633-
3874, Fax: +1-212-633-3820, and E-mail: reprints@elsevier.com.

Rheumatic Disease Clinics of North America is covered in *MEDLINE/PubMed (Index Medicus), Current
Contents/Clinical Medicine, Science Citation Index, ISI/BIOMED,* and *EMBASE/Excerpta Medica.*

Printed in the United States of America.

Health Disparities in Rheumatic Diseases: Part I

Editor

CANDACE H. FELDMAN

RHEUMATIC DISEASE CLINICS OF NORTH AMERICA

www.rheumatic.theclinics.com

Consulting Editor
MICHAEL H. WEISMAN

November 2020 • Volume 46 • Number 4

Contributors

CONSULTING EDITOR

MICHAEL H. WEISMAN, MD
Professor of Medicine, Emeritus, Division of Rheumatology, Cedars-Sinai Medical Center,
Distinguished Professor of Medicine, Emeritus, David Geffen School of Medicine,
University of California, Los Angeles, Los Angeles, California, USA

EDITOR

CANDACE H. FELDMAN, MD, MPH, ScD
Assistant Professor, Division of Rheumatology, Inflammation and Immunity, Department
of Medicine, Brigham and Women's Hospital, Harvard Medical School, Boston,
Massachusetts, USA

AUTHORS

ALLEN ANANDARAJAH, MD, MS
Professor of Medicine, Director, IQ Lupus Project, Division of Allergy, Immunology and
Rheumatology, University of Rochester Medical Center, Rochester, New York, USA

SHILPA ARORA, MD
Division of Rheumatology, Rush University Medical Center, Chicago, Illinois, USA

CHERYL BARNABE, MD, MSc, FRCPC
Associate Professor, Departments of Medicine, and Community Health Sciences,
Cumming School of Medicine, University of Calgary, Calgary, Alberta, Canada

YASHAAR CHAICHIAN, MD
Division of Immunology and Rheumatology, Department of Medicine, Stanford Medicine,
Stanford, California, USA

NICOLA DALBETH, MD, FRACP
Rheumatologist and Professor, Department of Medicine, Faculty of Medical and Health
Sciences, University of Auckland, Department of Rheumatology, Auckland District Health
Board, Auckland, New Zealand

KIMBERLY DEQUATTRO, MD, MM
Adjunct Instructor of Medicine, Division of Rheumatology, University of California, San
Francisco, San Francisco, California, USA

CRISTINA DRENKARD, MD, PhD
Associate Professor of Medicine and Epidemiology, Department of Medicine, Division of
Rheumatology, Emory University, Atlanta, Georgia, USA

TITILOLA FALASINNU, PhD
Departments of Epidemiology and Population Health, and Anesthesiology, Perioperative,
and Pain Medicine, Stanford Medicine, Stanford, California, USA

CANDACE H. FELDMAN, MD, MPH, ScD
Assistant Professor, Division of Rheumatology, Inflammation and Immunity, Department of Medicine, Brigham and Women's Hospital, Harvard Medical School, Boston, Massachusetts, USA

ELIZABETH D. FERUCCI, MD, MPH
Rheumatologist and Clinical Researcher, Division of Community Health Services, Department of Clinical and Research Services, Alaska Native Tribal Health Consortium, Anchorage, Alaska, USA

CHANDRA L. FORD, PhD, MPH, MLIS
Associate Professor, Department of Community Health Sciences, UCLA Fielding School of Public Health, University of California, Los Angeles, Los Angeles, California, USA

ANDREA GARCIA GUILLÉN, MD
Visiting Research Fellow, Department of Medicine, University of Auckland, Auckland, New Zealand

ANDREA M. KNIGHT, MD, MSCE
Division of Rheumatology, The Hospital for Sick Children, Toronto, Ontario, Canada

S. SAM LIM, MD, MPH
Professor of Medicine and Epidemiology, Department of Medicine, Division of Rheumatology, Emory University, Atlanta, Georgia, USA

DUNCAN F. MOORE, MD
Clinical Researcher, Division of Rheumatology, Department of Medicine, MedStar Georgetown University Hospital, Washington, DC, USA

MICHELLE MORSE, MD, MPH
Assistant Professor, Division of Global Health Equity, Department of Medicine, Brigham and Women's Hospital, Harvard Medical School, Boston, Massachusetts, USA

CHRISTINE A. PESCHKEN, MD, MSc, FRCPC
Associate Professor of Medicine and Community Health Sciences, Rady Faculty of Health Sciences, University of Manitoba, Winnipeg, Manitoba, Canada

TAMAR B. RUBINSTEIN, MD, MS
Department of Pediatrics, Division of Pediatric Rheumatology, Children's Hospital at Montefiore/Albert Einstein College of Medicine, Bronx, New York, USA

JULIA F. SIMARD, ScD
Department of Epidemiology and Population Health, Stanford Medicine, Division of Immunology and Rheumatology, Department of Medicine, Stanford Medicine, Stanford, California, USA

JASVINDER A. SINGH, MD, MPH
Rheumatologist and Professor, Medicine Service, VA Medical Center, Department of Medicine at the School of Medicine, Department of Epidemiology at the School of Public Health, The University of Alabama at Birmingham, Birmingham, Alabama, USA

VIRGINIA D. STEEN, MD
Division Chief, Division of Rheumatology, Department of Medicine, MedStar Georgetown University Hospital, Washington, DC, USA

LEANNE TE KARU, DipPharm, MHSc(Hons)
Prescribing Pharmacist, Ngā Kaitiaki o te Puna Rongoā o Aotearoa, Taupō, Associate Dean (Māori), School of Pharmacy, University of Otago, Dunedin, New Zealand

JESSICA N. WILLIAMS, MD, MPH
Rheumatology Fellow, Division of Rheumatology, Inflammation and Immunity, Department of Medicine, Brigham and Women's Hospital, Harvard Medical School, Boston, Massachusetts, USA

JINOOS YAZDANY, MD, MPH
Division of Rheumatology, University of California, San Francisco, San Francisco, California, USA

EDWARD YELIN, PhD
Emeritus Professor of Medicine and Health Policy, Division of Rheumatology and Philip R Lee Institute for Health Policy Studies, San Francisco, California, USA

Contents

I: Application of Theoretical Frameworks and Quality Metrics to Understand Rheumatic Disease Disparities

Jessica N. Williams, Chandra L. Ford, Michelle Morse, and Candace H. Feldman

> According to critical race theory (CRT), racism is ubiquitous in society. In the field of medicine, systems of racism are subtly interwoven with patient care, medical education, and medical research. Public health critical race praxis (PHCRP) is a tool that allows researchers to apply CRT to research. This article discusses the application of CRT and PHCRP to 3 race-related misconceptions in rheumatology: (1) giant cell arteritis is rare in non-white populations; (2) Black patients are less likely to undergo knee replacement because of patient preference; and (3) HLA-B*5801 screening should only be performed for patients of Asian descent.

S. Sam Lim and Cristina Drenkard

> Limitations in the ability to assemble large cohorts of patients with lupus from previously underrepresented groups have inhibited better understanding of many unanswered questions. The Georgians Organized Against Lupus (GOAL) Research Cohort is designed to overcome many of these limitations and is a rich and diverse repository of clinical, biological, sociodemographic, psychosocial, and health services data, and biologic material. Studies with the GOAL cohort will improve the understanding of how various factors interact and may lead to interventions on an individual and systems and societal level and help to mitigate the significant disparities that continue to exist in lupus.

Shilpa Arora and Jinoos Yazdany

> Assessment of quality of care for people with systemic lupus erythematosus (SLE) provides opportunities to identify gaps in health care and address disparities. Poor access to specialty care has been shown to negatively impact care in SLE and is associated with poor disease outcomes. Racial/ethnic minorities and those with low socioeconomic status are at higher risk for poor access and lower quality of care. Quality

measures evaluating processes of care have shown significant defi-
ciencies in care of SLE patients across studies. High SLE patient volume
correlates with better quality of care for providers in hospital and ambulatory settings.

Systemic lupus erythematosus (SLE) disproportionately affects those with
low socioeconomic status. Evidence from the past 2 decades has revealed
clearer distinctions on the mechanisms of poverty that affect long-term
outcomes in SLE. Poverty exacerbates direct, indirect, and humanistic
costs and is associated with worse SLE disease damage, greater mortality, and poorer quality of life. Ongoing commitments from medicine and society are required to reduce disparities, improve access to care, and
bolster resilience in persons with SLE who live in poverty.

II: Understanding Disease and Population-Specific Rheumatic Disease Disparities

Studies have described a high incidence and prevalence of several rheumatic diseases in indigenous North American populations. Conditions
studied most frequently with consistently high burden of disease include
rheumatoid arthritis, spondyloarthritis, and systemic lupus erythematosus.
Crystal-induced arthritis has been reported to have a lower prevalence
than expected. Information about genetic and environmental risk factors
is available for some of these conditions. An awareness of the epidemiology of rheumatic diseases in indigenous North American populations is
important for clinicians involved in caring for patients in these populations
as well as for planning health service delivery in these communities.

Disparities in prevalence, disease severity, physical and mental morbidity,
and mortality exist in childhood-onset systemic lupus (cSLE) that lead to
worse outcomes in children with systemic lupus erythematosus from socially disadvantaged backgrounds. Important gaps exist in knowledge
regarding many individual race/ethnicities across the globe, the interaction
between race/ethnicity and poverty, and drivers for identified disparities.
Large cSLE registries will facilitate investigating disparities in groups of patients that have yet to be identified. Social-ecological models can inform
approaches to investigate, monitor, and address disparities in cSLE.

Systemic lupus erythematosus (SLE) is a chronic multisystem autoimmune
disease characterized by autoantibody production and diverse clinical
manifestations. The many complex, overlapping, and closely associated

factors that influence SLE susceptibility and outcomes include ethnic disparities, low adherence to medications, and poverty, and geography. Epigenetic mechanisms may provide the link between these environmental exposures and behaviors and the disproportionate burden of SLE seen in ethnic minorities. Attention to these modifiable social determinants of health would not only improve outcomes for vulnerable patients with SLE but likely reduce susceptibility to SLE as well through epigenetic changes.

Proximal, intermediate, and distal social determinants of health inform the health of populations. Differences in rheumatoid arthritis outcomes between populations reflect inequities in these determinants. However, health service access, medication availability, and high-quality care interactions can be ensured through health system restructuring and innovations in individual-level care provision. This article summarizes disparities in rheumatoid arthritis care that have been recognized and described in the United States and Canada and proposes models of care and treatment approaches that can support better outcomes for population groups at risk for outcome inequities.

Although effective and low-cost urate-lowering therapy has been available for decades, inequities in gout management exist. Despite high impact of disease, rates of urate-lowering therapy prescription are low in women, in African-Americans in the United States, in Māori (Indigenous New Zealanders), and in Pacific peoples living in Aotearoa/New Zealand. Social determinants of health, barriers to accessing the health care system, health literacy demands, stigmatization, and bias contribute to inequities in gout burden and management. Approaches that focus on building health literacy and delivering culturally safe care lead to improved outcomes in gout, and offer important solutions to achieve health equity.

Racial and ethnic disparities in systemic sclerosis are abundant. The incidence, severity of end-organ manifestations, functional impairment, quality of life, and mortality of systemic sclerosis vary by ethnic group. This article summarizes such disparities and explores the role of socioeconomic status in their development and persistence.

Significant disparities exist in systemic lupus erythematosus (SLE) regarding prevalence, disease severity, and mortality, with race/ethnic minorities being disproportionately affected in the United States. This review highlights that despite these disparities, race/ethnic minority under-representation remains an issue within SLE research. Decreased race/ethnic minority involvement in SLE research has real-world implications, including less understanding of the disease and less applicability of approved therapies among diverse groups of patients. Members of the SLE research community have an obligation to narrow this gap to ensure that future advances within the field are derived from and benefit a more representative group of patients.

Designing an Intervention to Improve Management of High-Risk Lupus Patients Through Care Coordination   723

Allen Anandarajah

Health care disparities are a major cause for large discrepancies in health outcomes between different populations with systemic lupus erythematosus in the United States.A team-based model that incorporates a care co-ordination strategy in the management of high-risk lupus patients can provide an effective method to overcome the obstacles posed by health care disparities.Access, behavioral modification, community outreach programs, depression, and education are key aspects that need to be addressed when designing interventions to improve the quality of care for high-risk lupus patients.

RHEUMATIC DISEASE CLINICS
OF NORTH AMERICA

SERIES OF RELATED INTEREST

Medical Clinics of North America
https://www.medical.theclinics.com/
Neurologic Clinics
https://www.neurologic.theclinics.com/
Dermatologic Clinics
https://www.derm.theclinics.com/
Physical Medicine and Rehabilitation Clinics of North America
https://www.pmr.theclinics.com/

THE CLINICS ARE AVAILABLE ONLINE!
Access your subscription at:
www.theclinics.com

Foreword

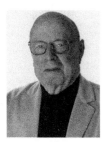

Michael H. Weisman, MD
Consulting Editor

Candace Feldman has taken on the task of assembling information for Rheumatologists that address health disparities in our rheumatic diseases. This is a very large topic and we will approach it in two separate Clinics issues; each will address the concept that racial bias is embedded in all aspects of society, affecting rheumatologic care of individual patients, education of our trainees, and most importantly, research design and interpretation. For the current volume, Sam Lim and Christina Drenkard discuss the importance of including social determinants of health within the framework of large data collections intended to ask research questions; Arora and Yazdany address many of the reasons why poor access to specialty care afflict the systemic lupus erythematosus (SLE) community and why quality measures are useful as research tools to identify these gaps. De Quattro and Yelin tackle the issue of residence in areas of concentrated poverty as primary reasons why individuals with SLE have severe negative health outcomes; Cheryl Barnabe points out why adherence to quality-of-care indicators and patient experience in rheumatology care can close gaps in the highly variable care delivered to rheumatoid arthritis patients today. Liz Ferucci notes the excessive burden of rheumatic diseases experienced by indigenous North American populations and how the understudied areas of epidemiology, genetics, and environmental risk contribute to this burden. Rubenstein and Knight highlight the fact that childhood-onset SLE is clearly understudied in terms of our appreciation for the health inequities present in this special population.

Guillen and colleagues address the underappreciated area of disparities in gout burden and its management that occur across the world; health literacy and cultural understanding impose major barriers to effective gout management, and these must be addressed by health organizations and systems. Moore and Steen point out the understudied areas of health inequities in both incidence and severity of systemic sclerosis, focusing on the possibility that more equitable access to care might close the gaps in this disease. The final 3 articles in this remarkable collection address SLE disparities in a fine-tuned way: Peschkin points out how mistrust and poor communication contribute to worse outcomes in nonwhite ethnicities and how hazardous environmental exposures contribute to risk; Falasinnu and colleagues at Stanford discuss

https://doi.org/10.1016/j.rdc.2020.08.002
0889-857X/20/© 2020 Published by Elsevier Inc.
rheumatic.theclinics.com

how inadequate inclusion of race/ethnic minorities in SLE clinical trials contribute to our lack of understanding of the heterogeneous responses to treatment interventions; and Anandarajah identifies for us the importance of a team approach to care coordination strategies for SLE patients where depression and education inequities clearly affect the quality of care for SLE patients.

This issue is incredibly timely and important as we all are confronting the explicit and implicit biases in ourselves and our institutions. The downstream effect of these feelings, emotions, and actions in the world of Rheumatology are given a strong boost to be placed on the front burner of our conduct. Dr Feldman has done a remarkable job.

Michael H. Weisman, MD
Division of Rheumatology
Cedars–Sinai Medical Center
David Geffen School of Medicine at
University of California, Los Angeles
1545 Calmar Court
Los Angeles, CA 90024, USA

E-mail address:
michael.weisman@cshs.org

Preface

Issue 1

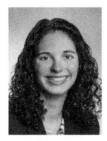

Candace H. Feldman, MD, MPH, ScD
Editor

A health disparity is defined as "a health difference that is closely linked with social, economic, and/or environmental disadvantage."[1] Specifically, disparities result in a disproportionate burden of disease and of potentially avoidable adverse outcomes among groups of individuals who have systematically and oftentimes deliberately been forced to experience barriers to achieving health and high-quality health care. Disparities may be observed by "any characteristic historically linked to discrimination or exclusion," including but not limited to race/ethnicity, socioeconomic status, religion, sexual orientation, gender identity, age, geographic location, or disability.[1]

In this first issue, authors describe the myriad of ways in which disparities adversely affect individuals with chronic rheumatic diseases. Two frameworks: Critical race theory and Social determinants of health, are presented to guide the way disparities are studied, described, and ultimately how they may be addressed. Critical race theory asserts that race is a social construct and highlights the pervasive role racism continues to play in our society and in health care.[2] Social determinants of health refer to the "features of and pathways by which societal conditions affect health and that potentially can be altered by informed action."[3] Studies demonstrating the role of socioeconomic status both at the individual and at the area levels are clear applications of the way in which social determinants directly influence health outcomes. Within the health care setting, the use of quality metrics is described as another potential strategy to guide both the way in which disparities are documented and how they may be addressed. This issue also explores disease-specific disparities by factors including race/ethnicity, gender, and region in rheumatoid arthritis, systemic lupus erythematosus, systemic sclerosis, and gout. Authors also describe population-specific disparities in childhood-onset lupus, and among the American Indian/Alaska Native populations.

Rheum Dis Clin N Am 46 (2020) xv–xvi
https://doi.org/10.1016/j.rdc.2020.08.001
0889-857X/20/© 2020 Published by Elsevier Inc.
rheumatic.theclinics.com

In this issue, we present the striking prevalence of health disparities in the field of rheumatology. The COVID-19 pandemic has further revealed and deepened existing disparities by race/ethnicity and socioeconomic status that require urgent multifaceted, multilevel interventions by our rheumatology community. We offer frameworks to consider these disparities and the impetus to address them through further research, high-quality patient care, and advocacy.

Candace H. Feldman, MD, MPH, ScD
Division of Rheumatology, Inflammation
and Immunity
Brigham and Women's Hospital
Harvard Medical School
60 Fenwood Road
Boston, MA 02115, USA

E-mail address:
cfeldman@bwh.harvard.edu

REFERENCES

1. The Secretary's Advisory Committee on National Health Promotion and Disease Prevention Objectives for 2020. In: Department of Health and Human Services, editor. Phase I report: recommendations for the framework and format of Healthy People 2020. Washington, DC; 2010. Available at: http://www.healthypeople.gov/sites/default/files/PhaseI_0.pdf.
2. Ford CL, Airhihenbuwa CO. Critical Race Theory, race equity, and public health: toward antiracism praxis. Am J Public Health 2010;100(suppl 1):S30–5.
3. Krieger N. A glossary for social epidemiology. J Epidemiol Community Health 2001;55(10):693–700.

I. Application of Theoretical Frameworks and Quality Metrics to Understand Rheumatic Disease Disparities

Racial Disparities in Rheumatology Through the Lens of Critical Race Theory

Jessica N. Williams, MD, MPH[a],*, Chandra L. Ford, PhD, MPH, MLIS[b],
Michelle Morse, MD, MPH[c], Candace H. Feldman, MD, MPH, ScD[d]

KEYWORDS

• Race • Disparities • Giant cell arteritis • Osteoarthritis • Gout

KEY POINTS

• Race is a social construct, and there is considerable ancestral heterogeneity within racial groups.

• Critical race theory asserts that racism remains pervasive in society. The authors propose applying this theory to better understand and address racial/ethnic disparities in rheumatic diseases using the public health critical race praxis.

• Contrary to traditional teaching, giant cell arteritis is not rare in non-White populations, which often have considerable White ancestry.

• Lower rates of knee arthroplasties among Black patients cannot be fully attributed to patient preference; physicians must appropriately educate and build trust with patients and examine their own biases.

• HLA-B*5801 allele frequency and allopurinol-associated severe cutaneous adverse reactions remain elevated among Black patients but few rheumatologists order testing; thus, this population may benefit from genetic screening.

INTRODUCTION

The term race has historically been defined as a distinct group of people with similar physical characteristics and ancestry.[1] However, the work of late 20th century

Funding source: Brigham and Women's Hospital Health Equity Innovation Pilot Grant.
[a] Division of Rheumatology, Inflammation and Immunity, Department of Medicine, Brigham and Women's Hospital, Harvard Medical School, 60 Fenwood Road, Boston, MA 02115, USA; [b] Department of Community Health Sciences, Jonathan & Karin Fielding School of Public Health, University of California at Los Angeles, Box 951772, 650 Charles East Young Drive, South, Los Angeles, CA 90095-1772, USA; [c] Division of Global Health Equity, Department of Medicine, Brigham and Women's Hospital, Harvard Medical School, 75 Francis Street, Boston, MA 02115, USA; [d] Division of Rheumatology, Inflammation and Immunity, Department of Medicine, Brigham and Women's Hospital, Harvard Medical School, 60 Fenwood Road, Office #6016P, Boston, MA 02115, USA
* Corresponding author.
E-mail address: jwilliams62@bwh.harvard.edu

geneticists has confirmed that race is not a biologic construct based on genetics, but rather a social construct invented by those who would classify themselves as White in order to subjugate members of other races.[1] Indeed, geneticists and paleontologists have demonstrated that all human beings have ancestral origin in Africa,[2] and that there is more ancestral diversity within racial groups than between racial groups.[3] White race is often considered to be an exclusive group of pure European origin, and individuals who have a White parent and a non-White parent are typically assigned to the non-White group because of this concept of hypodescent.[4] Historically within the United States, the dominant narrative was that lighter skin color and ancestral European origin (also known as White race) was superior to darker skin color and ancestral origin in Africa, Asia, or the Americas.[5] This notion of White supremacy suggested that members of the White race were physically, intellectually, and morally superior to darker-skinned people. In the United States, this narrative of White supremacy was used to justify the genocide and theft of property from American Indians, the brutal enslavement and subsequent multifaceted oppression of Black Americans, and the discrimination against and marginalization of Asian American and Hispanic American communities. Consequences of this White supremacist ideology reverberate to this day, with ongoing massive inequality between the races in regards to wealth accrual, employment opportunities, incarceration rates, health care access and outcomes, and many other measures.[6] This enforced racial hierarchy, which has historically been perpetuated by the US government in order to uplift members of the White race, is also known as racism.[7]

In order to better study and combat the nuanced ways racism operates in the post-civil rights era, critical race theory (CRT) was formulated by a group of non-White legal scholars in 1989,[8] with foundations in the work of Derrick Bell.[9,10] According to CRT, racism is pervasive in modern US society, and is often covert. In regards to medicine and public health, CRT asserts that racism itself is a social determinant of health, and that racial bias has been incorporated into medical knowledge in ways that reinforce White supremacy. CRT has been applied to the field of health equity research using the public health critical race praxis (PHCRP),[11] which provides guidance for biomedical researchers (Fig. 1). The PHCRP framework considers all research to be informed by a priori biases; therefore, it calls for critical examination of a priori assumptions related to racial issues. In addition, it considers the complex ways in which membership in multiple oppressed groups may affect individuals synergistically (a concept known as intersectionality), the need for the perspectives of marginalized groups to drive the research process, and the need to take action based on the research outcome in order to advance racial health equity.

This article applies the PHCRP version of CRT to race-related topics in rheumatology. Many rheumatic diseases are associated with known racial and ethnic disparities,[12,13] which are defined by the Institute of Medicine as "differences in the quality of care received by minorities and non-minorities who have equal access to care... when there are no differences between these groups in their preferences and needs for treatment."[14] Specifically, the article explores three common misconceptions among rheumatologists through the lens of CRT:

Giant cell arteritis is rare in non-White populations.
Black patients are less likely to undergo knee replacement surgery because of patient preference.
HLA-B*5801 screening should only be performed for patients of Asian descent.

Accordingly, this article will explore how racism, racial bias, and lack of understanding of ancestral heterogeneity within racial groups perpetuate these common rheumatologic myths.

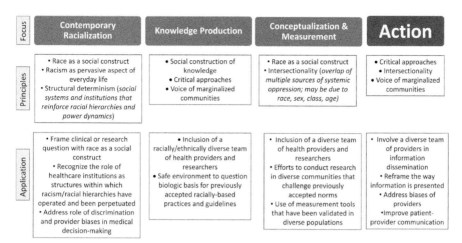

Fig. 1. Public health critical race praxis. (*Data from* Ford CL, Airhihenbuwa CO. The public health critical race methodology: praxis for antiracism research. Soc Sci Med 2010;71:1390-8; and Ford CL, Airhihenbuwa CO. Critical race theory, race equity, and public health: toward antiracism praxis. Am J Public Health 2010;100 Suppl 1:S30-5.)

CONTENT

Myth 1: Giant Cell Arteritis is Rare in Non-White Populations

Giant cell arteritis (GCA), the most common type of systemic vasculitis, may lead to adverse outcomes such as blindness and stroke if not diagnosed and treated promptly.[15] The incidence of GCA was initially studied in predominantly White populations of northern European ancestry who were at increased risk for this disease,[16] and historically GCA was believed to be exceedingly rare in non-White populations. For example, GCA has been found to be two- to fivefold more common in northern European versus southern European countries.[17] Compared with White Americans, the risk of GCA has historically been reported to be 20 times lower in Asian Americans, five to seven times lower in Black Americans, and lower in Hispanic-Americans and people of Arabic descent.[17] However, more recent studies have found that GCA is not as rare among non-White populations in the United States as was previously thought. A 2019 study from the Johns Hopkins Wilmer Eye Institute found that among 92 patients over the age of 50 with biopsy-proven GCA treated between 2007 and 2017, 15% self-identified as Black.[18] In that study, there was no significant difference in the incidence rate of biopsy-proven GCA between White and Black patients (incidence rate ratio 1.2; 95% confidence interval [CI] 0.6–2.4; $P=.66$). Similarly, a study of 32 patients with biopsy-proven GCA treated at the University of Miami between 1996 and 2002 found that 41% of these patients self-identified as Hispanic.[19] As these studies have demonstrated, GCA is not rare in non-White populations, and rheumatologists must maintain a high level of vigilance in order to detect and treat all patients with GCA in a timely manner, regardless of their race or ethnicity.

This controversy regarding race and GCA emphasizes an important concept, the ancestral heterogeneity within racial groups in the US. For example, Americans who self-identify as Black have 24% genome-wide European ancestry on average.[20] The European ancestry among Black American descendants of slaves is attributable to widespread rape of Black women by White men during slavery[21] and consensual inter-racial relationships since the mid-20th century. Additionally, Hispanic Americans frequently have mixed European, Native American, and/or African ancestry; the average amount of genome-wide European ancestry among Hispanic Americans is 65%.[20] It is important for physicians, including rheumatologists, to understand this ancestral heterogeneity in order to avoid making incorrect assumptions regarding disease risk based on a patient's assumed or self-reported race. Indeed, this sort of diagnostic triage based on race may lead to missed diagnoses, untreated disease, and avoidable adverse outcomes that contribute further to racial inequities.

Myth 2: Black Patients Are Less Likely to Undergo Knee Replacement Surgery Due to Patient Preference

Osteoarthritis (OA) is the most common type of arthritis globally, with over 80% of cases involving the knee.[22] The only curative treatment for knee OA is knee replacement surgery, or knee arthroplasty. Several studies have demonstrated that in the United States, Black patients have lower rates of knee arthroplasty than White patients.[23–29] US nationwide studies have also shown that economic factors do not explain the lower odds of knee arthroplasty in Black men.[24,30] Other studies have reported that Black patients are less willing to undergo joint replacement surgery because of lack of understanding of the procedure, concerns about procedure efficacy, increased perception of operative risk, and concerns about postoperative pain and debilitation.[31–35] Additional studies have reported that when Black patients are given a hypothetical scenario between medical versus surgical treatment of knee OA, they are less likely to choose surgery (odds ratio [OR] 0.63, 95% CI 0.42–0.93),[36] and that racial differences in patient preference for total joint replacement may fully explain known racial disparities in joint replacement rates.[37]

However, attributing this racial disparity in knee arthroplasty rates to patient preference ignores both the responsibility of physicians to fully educate all patients about the risks and benefits of knee arthroplasty using nontechnical language that is tailored to an individual patient's health literacy, as well as the ways that provider characteristics (eg, implicit bias) may contribute. Studies have found that videos that educate Black patients about knee arthroplasty can improve expectations about the postoperative course[38] and that increased knowledge about knee arthroplasty among minorities can mitigate racial disparities in receipt of this procedure.[39] Additionally, mistrust of physicians may influence Black patients' decisions regarding knee arthroplasty. It is the physician's responsibility to build rapport with patients of color, particularly given the history of mistreatment of communities of color by the US medical establishment, which has engendered this mistrust. Black patients have been found to have worse outcomes than White patients after joint replacement surgery,[40] possibly related to delayed care/more advanced disease at presentation or poorer quality of care; it is therefore conceivable that Black patients know individuals within their social networks who have had poor outcomes after joint replacement, which may discourage receipt of surgery. Lastly, physicians have an obligation to be aware of their own racial biases, which may affect how patients are counseled about knee arthroplasty. For example, a 2014 study presented 543 primary care physicians (PCPs) with a hypothetical scenario describing either a Black or White patient with severe OA refractory to medical treatment, and found that PCPs had significant implicit and explicit racial bias that led them to label White patients as more medically cooperative, which could conceivably affect referral patterns for knee arthroplasty.[41] In summary, patient preference regarding knee arthroplasty can only be determined after physicians have educated patients about the risks and benefits of the surgery using appropriate language, established a trusting relationship with patients, and accounted for the racial and other biases they bring to the clinical encounter.

*Myth 3: HLA-B*5801 Screening Should Only Be Performed for Patients of Asian Descent*

Gout is an episodic arthritis that affects greater than 3% of the US population,[42] and the first-line treatment is the urate-lowering drug allopurinol. The most feared complications of allopurinol are severe cutaneous adverse reaction (SCARs), which may be fatal in up to 25% of cases.[43] The risk of allopurinol-associated SCARs in the general population is low at 0.1% to 0.4%; however, risk increases by greater than 500-fold in individuals who possess the HLA-B*5801 allele.[43] The 2012 American College of Rheumatology (ACR) guidelines for the management of gout recommend screening for the HLA-B*5801 allele prior to initiation of allopurinol in several populations of East Asian descent (Koreans with $\geq$ stage III chronic kidney disease, Han Chinese, and Thai).[44] This recommendation is based on literature revealing that HLA-B*5801 allele frequency is increased in these populations (6%–12%), along with greater than 300-fold increased risk of SCARs in these populations when exposed to allopurinol.[45–47]

However, the frequency of the HLA-B*5801 allele is also higher in Black patients (4%–6%) compared with White and Hispanic patients (both 1%).[48] Additionally, a 2018 US Medicaid study found that both Black and Asian patients have a threefold higher risk of allopurinol-associated SCARs compared with White and Hispanic patients.[49] The 2020 American College of Rheumatology guidelines update the conditional recommendation for HLA-B*5801 testing and now include Black individuals with patients of Southeast Asian descent.[50] However, currently rheumatologists are not trained to routinely screen Black patients for HLA-B*5801 positivity prior to initiating allopurinol, even though the consequences of not screening may be life-threatening. It is also important to recognize the constraints of using race to classify patients, as patients' genetic makeup may not be reflected by their apparent or self-reported race.

SUMMARY

CRT provides rheumatologists with a framework to study racial disparities related to rheumatic diseases and clarify exactly how racism contributes to them. One needs to understand that racism and racial bias are deeply embedded in all aspects of society; rheumatologic patient care, education, and research are not excepted. This article draws on CRT in order to offer guidance regarding 3 problems in the area of rheumatic disease that warrant further attention. Rheumatologists are taught that GCA is rare in non-White populations, even though recent studies have disputed this dogma; this example highlights that non-White populations may actually have considerable amounts of White ancestry, and that physicians are potentially misdiagnosing non-White patients with GCA, which may lead to serious consequences such as preventable blindness. Physicians are taught that Black patients with advanced, medically refractory osteoarthritis choose not to have total knee arthroplasties; however, this assertion is based on incomplete data, which neither account for the responsibility physicians have to educate their patients and build trusting relationships with them, nor examine how phsycians' own racial biases may affect the way they care for and counsel patients. Physicians are taught that they should screen patients of Korean, Han Chinese, and Thai descent for HLA-B*5801 prior to initiation of allopurinol for treatment of gout, but have not been taught do so for Black patients even though they too have significantly elevated risk of carrying the HLA-B*5801 allele and suffering from allopurinol-associated SCARs. CRT teaches that one must continually examine the field's beliefs in regard to race-related topics so that one is promoting health equity for all and taking the best possible care of one's patients.

DISCLOSURE

The authors have nothing to disclose.

REFERENCES

1. Takezawa YI, Smedley A, Wade P. Race. In: Encyclopaedia Britannica. 2020. Available at: https://www.britannica.com/topic/race-human. Accessed February 3, 2020.
2. Hublin J-J, Ben-Ncer A, Bailey SE, et al. New fossils from Jebel Irhoud, Morocco and the pan-African origin of Homo sapiens. Nature 2017;546:289–92.
3. Lewontin RC. The apportionment of human diversity. In: Dobzhansky TH, Hecht MK, Steere WC, editors. Evolutionary biology. New York: Springer; 1972. p. 381–98.
4. Peery D, Bodenhausen GV. Black + white = black: hypodescent in reflexive categorization of racially ambiguous faces. Psychol Sci 2008;19:973–7.
5. Fredrickson G. White supremacy. Oxford: Oxford University Press; 1981.
6. Hanks A, Solomon D, Weller CE. Systematic inequality. In: Center for American Progress. 2018. Available at: https://www.americanprogress.org/issues/race/reports/2018/02/21/447051/systematic-inequality/. Accessed February 4, 2020.
7. Smedley A. Racism. In: Encyclopaedia Britannica. 2017. Available at: https://www.britannica.com/topic/racism. Accessed February 4, 2020.
8. Ford CL, Airhihenbuwa CO. Critical race theory, race equity, and public health: toward antiracism praxis. Am J Public Health 2010;100(Suppl 1):S30–5.
9. Bell D. Race, racism, and American law. Boston: Little, Brown; 1973.
10. Bell D. Faces at the bottom of the well: the permanence of racism. New York: Basic Books; 1992.
11. Ford CL, Airhihenbuwa CO. The public health critical race methodology: praxis for antiracism research. Soc Sci Med 2010;71:1390–8.
12. Greenberg JD, Spruill TM, Shan Y, et al. Racial and ethnic disparities in disease activity in rheumatoid arthritis patients. Am J Med 2013;126:1089–98.
13. Somers EC, Marder W, Cagnoli P, et al. Population-based incidence and prevalence of systemic lupus erythematosus: The Michigan Lupus Epidemiology and Surveillance Program. Arthritis Rheumatol 2014;66:369–78.
14. Smedley BD, Stith AY, Nelson AR. Unequal treatment: confronting racial and ethnic disparities in health care. Washington, DC: National Academies Press; 2003.
15. Berti A, Dejaco C. Update on the epidemiology, risk factors, and outcomes of systemic vasculitides. Best Pract Res Clin Rheumatol 2018;32:271–94.
16. Chandran AK, Udayakumar PD, Crowson CS, et al. The incidence of giant cell arteritis in Olmsted County, Minnesota, over a 60-year period 1950-2009. Scand J Rheumatol 2015;44:215–8.
17. Piram M, Maldini C, Mahr A. Effect of race/ethnicity on risk, presentation and course of connective tissue diseases and primary systemic vasculitides. Curr Opin Rheumatol 2012;24:193–200.
18. Gruener AM, Poostchi A, Carey AR, et al. Association of giant cell arteritis with race. JAMA Ophthalmol 2019.
19. Lam BL, Wirthlin RS, Gonzalez A, et al. Giant cell arteritis among Hispanic Americans. Am J Ophthalmol 2007;143:161–3.
20. Bryc K, Durand EY, Macpherson JM, et al. The genetic ancestry of African Americans, Latinos, and European Americans across the United States. Am J Hum Genet 2015;96:37–53.

21. Moon D. Slavery. In: Smith MD, editor. Encyclopedia of rape. Westport (CT): Greenwood; 2004. p. 235.

22. Vos T, Flaxman AD, Naghavi M, et al. Years lived with disability (YLDs) for 1160 sequelae of 289 diseases and injuries 1990-2010: a systematic analysis for the Global Burden of Disease Study 2010. Lancet 2012;380:2163-96.

23. Skinner J, Weinstein JN, Sporer SM, et al. Racial, ethnic, and geographic disparities in rates of knee arthroplasty among Medicare patients. N Engl J Med 2003; 349:1350-9.

24. Skinner J, Zhou W, Weinstein J. The influence of income and race on total knee arthroplasty in the United States. J Bone Joint Surg Am 2006;88:2159-66.

25. Centers for Disease Control and Prevention (CDC). Racial disparities in total knee replacement among Medicare enrollees–United States, 2000-2006. MMWR Morb Mortal Wkly Rep 2009;58:133-8.

26. Singh JA, Lu X, Rosenthal GE, et al. Racial disparities in knee and hip total joint arthroplasty: an 18-year analysis of national Medicare data. Ann Rheum Dis 2014; 73:2107-15.

27. Zhang W, Lyman S, Boutin-Foster C, et al. Racial and ethnic disparities in utilization rate, hospital volume, and perioperative outcomes after total knee arthroplasty. J Bone Joint Surg Am 2016;98:1243-52.

28. MacFarlane LA, Kim E, Cook NR, et al. Racial variation in total knee replacement in a diverse nationwide clinical trial. J Clin Rheumatol 2018;24:1-5.

29. Cavanaugh AM, Rauh MJ, Thompson CA, et al. Racial and ethnic disparities in utilization of total knee arthroplasty among older women. Osteoarthr Cartil 2019;27:1746-54.

30. Hanchate AD, Zhang Y, Felson DT, et al. Exploring the determinants of racial and ethnic disparities in total knee arthroplasty: health insurance, income, and assets. Med Care 2008;46:481-8.

31. Ibrahim SA, Siminoff LA, Burant CJ, et al. Variations in perceptions of treatment and self-care practices in elderly with osteoarthritis: a comparison between African American and white patients. Arthritis Rheum 2001;45:340-5.

32. Ibrahim SA, Siminoff LA, Burant CJ, et al. Understanding ethnic differences in the utilization of joint replacement for osteoarthritis. Med Care 2002;40(Suppl 1):1-44.

33. Ibrahim SA, Siminoff LA, Burant CJ, et al. Differences in expectations of outcome mediate African American/white patient differences in "willingness" to consider joint replacement. Arthritis Rheum 2002;46:2429-35.

34. Lavernia CJ, Alcerro JC, Rossi MD. Fear in arthroplasty surgery: the role of race. Clin Orthop Relat Res 2010;468:547-54.

35. Gandhi R, Razak F, Davey JR, et al. Ethnicity and patient's perception of risk in joint replacement surgery. J Rheumatol 2008;35:1664-7.

36. Byrne MM, Souchek J, Richardson M, et al. Racial/ethnic differences in preferences for total knee replacement surgery. J Clin Epidemiol 2006;59:1078-86.

37. Hausmann LR, Mor M, Hanusa BH, et al. The effect of patient race on total joint replacement recommendations and utilization in the orthopedic setting. J Gen Intern Med 2010;25:982-8.

38. Weng HH, Kaplan RM, Boscardin WJ, et al. Development of a decision aid to address racial disparities in utilization of knee replacement surgery. Arthritis Rheum 2007;57:568-75.

39. Kwoh CK, Vina ER, Cloonan YK, et al. Determinants of patient preferences for total knee replacement: African-Americans and whites. Arthritis Res Ther 2015; 17:348.

40. Stone AH, MacDonald JH, Joshi MS, et al. Differences in perioperative outcomes and complications between African American and white patients after total joint arthroplasty. J Arthroplasty 2019;34:656–62.

41. Oliver MN, Wells KM, Joy-Gaba JA, et al. Do physicians' implicit views of African Americans affect clinical decision making? J Am Board Fam Med 2014;27: 177–88.

42. Juraschek SP, Miller ER 3rd, Gelber AC. Body mass index, obesity, and prevalent gout in the United States in 1988-1994 and 2007-2010. Arthritis Care Res (Hoboken) 2013;65:127–32.

43. Hershfield MS, Callaghan JT, Tassaneeyakul W, et al. Clinical Pharmacogenetics Implementation Consortium guidelines for human leukocyte antigen-B genotype and allopurinol dosing. Clin Pharmacol Ther 2013;93:153–8.

44. Khanna D, Fitzgerald JD, Khanna PP, et al. 2012 American College of Rheumatology guidelines for management of gout. Part 1: systematic nonpharmacologic and pharmacologic therapeutic approaches to hyperuricemia. Arthritis Care Res (Hoboken) 2012;64:1431–46.

45. Jung JW, Song WJ, Kim YS, et al. HLA-B58 can help the clinical decision on starting allopurinol in patients with chronic renal insufficiency. Nephrol Dial Transplant 2011;26:3567–72.

46. Hung SI, Chung WH, Liou LB, et al. HLA-B*5801 allele as a genetic marker for severe cutaneous adverse reactions caused by allopurinol. Proc Natl Acad Sci U S A 2005;102:4134–9.

47. Tassaneeyakul W, Jantararoungtong T, Chen P, et al. Strong association between HLA-B*5801 and allopurinol-induced Stevens-Johnson syndrome and toxic epidermal necrolysis in a Thai population. Pharmacogenet Genomics 2009;19: 704–9.

48. Ford S, Kimball P, Gupta G, et al. HLA-B*58:01 genotype and the risk of allopurinol-associated severe cutaneous adverse reactions in a predominately black or African American population with advanced chronic kidney disease [abstract]. Arthritis Rheumatol 2018;70(suppl 10). Available at: https://acrabstracts. org/abstract/hla-b5801-genotype-and-the-risk-of-allopurinol-associated-severe-cutaneous-adverse-reactions-in-a-predominately-black-or-african-american-population-with-advanced-chronic-kidney-disease/. Accessed July 28, 2020.

49. Keller SF, Lu N, Blumenthal KG, et al. Racial/ethnic variation and risk factors for allopurinol-associated severe cutaneous adverse reactions: a cohort study. Ann Rheum Dis 2018;77:1187–93.

50. FitzGerald JD, Dalbeth N, Mikuls T et al. 2020 American College of Rheumatology Guideline for the Management of Gout. Arthritis Care & Resaerch Vol 0, No 0 June 2020 pp 1-17).

Understanding Lupus Disparities Through a Social Determinants of Health Framework

The Georgians Organized Against Lupus Research Cohort

S. Sam Lim, MD, MPH*, Cristina Drenkard, MD, PhD

KEYWORDS

• Systemic lupus erythematosus • Social determinants of health • Disparities

KEY POINTS

- Limitations in the ability to assemble large cohorts of patients with lupus from previously underrepresented groups have been a significant barrier to better understanding many unanswered questions.
- Including social determinants in the health disparities framework provides a more comprehensive understanding of the reasons why communities of color experience disparities in disease burden and outcome.
- The GOAL research cohort is a repository of diverse data and biologic material that will improve the understanding of how social determinants impact lupus.

DISPARITIES IN LUPUS

As recently as the early 1950s, systemic lupus erythematosus (SLE) was felt to have a strong predilection for females of childbearing age, be associated with some drugs, and have a genetic component. At the time, there was relatively little attention to race, with the distribution of disease in the population being felt to be proportionate to the population under care at that time, which were mostly females with light hair, fair skin, and an inability to tan.[1,2] The first major population-based study of SLE in the United States, published in 1970, uncovered the striking racial/ethnic disparities in disease distribution

Department of Medicine, Division of Rheumatology, Emory University, 49 Jesse Hill Jr. Drive, Southeast, Atlanta, GA 30303, USA
* Corresponding author.
E-mail address: sslim@emory.edu
Twitter: @LupusDocLim (S.S.L.)

Rheum Dis Clin N Am 46 (2020) 613–621
https://doi.org/10.1016/j.rdc.2020.07.002
0889-857X/20/© 2020 Elsevier Inc. All rights reserved.
rheumatic.theclinics.com

that are acknowledged today.[3] Subsequently, there has also been increased recognition of the disparities in the onset, acuity, and outcomes from different ethnic groups. Patients from racial minorities are more likely to suffer from multiple comorbidities; they have a higher prevalence of depression, cardiovascular disease (CVD), and diabetes, and worse health-related quality of life (HRQL) than whites.[4–10]

THE LEGACY OF LUpus in MInorities: NAture versus Nurture

In 1994, Dr. Graciela Alarcón from the University of Alabama at Birmingham (UAB) led a study to better understand the relationship of ethnicity to SLE outcomes. Patients of Hispanic, African American, and Caucasian ancestry were recruited from 3 sites: UAB, the University of Texas Health Science Center at Houston, and the University of Puerto Rico. The study, aptly named LUpus in MInorities: NAture versus Nurture (LUMINA), was comprised of 234 African Americans, 220 Hispanic, and 181 Caucasian patients. Over the years, LUMINA has contributed extensively to the SLE disparities literature through numerous articles, abstracts, and other publications. LUMINA highlighted many disparities (and associated factors) disproportionately afflicting Hispanics and African Americans with SLE compared with their Caucasian counterparts, including more renal involvement (ancestral genes ± socioeconomic factors), increased disease activity (ethnicity early but not later in the disease), diminished survival (poverty), and more adverse pregnancy outcomes (socioeconomic factors).[11]

The LUMINA study was a harbinger of growing evidence suggesting that most health problems occur long before people get to their health care provider, with medical care contributing only partially to the overall health status of the population. Thus, given the nature of disparities, interventions are needed within and outside the health care system. Effective efforts to improve health and reduce gaps in health need to pay greater attention to addressing the nonmedical determinants of health. A critical mass of relevant knowledge has accumulated, documenting associations, exploring pathways and biological mechanisms, and providing a previously unavailable scientific foundation for appreciating the role of social factors in health. US public health leaders and researchers have increasingly recognized that the dramatic health problems people face cannot be successfully addressed by medical care alone.

SOCIAL DETERMINANTS OF HEALTH

Historically, many public health efforts have focused primarily on individual behaviors. Social determinants of health (SDH) are conditions in the environments in which people are born, live, learn, work, play, worship, and age that affect a wide range of health, functioning, and quality-of-life outcomes and risks. Including social determinants in the health disparities framework provides a more comprehensive understanding of the reasons why low-income communities and communities of color experience disproportionately higher rates of disease, health care utilization, and death. These conditions shape people's options, choice, and behavior, which can then in turn impact outcomes. Studies of social determinants have been relatively lacking and are imperative in SLE, where the disease disproportionately impacts minority communities, and biologic factors cannot fully explain or address health disparities.

THE GEORGIA LUPUS REGISTRY

Limitations in the ability to assemble large population-based cohorts of patients with systemic and/or cutaneous lupus with validated diagnoses and with significant representation from previously under-represented sociodemographic groups have been a significant barrier to better understanding the true clinical burden of lupus, as well as the many unanswered questions related to treatment, health care access, and natural history. Furthermore, it is also challenging and expensive to follow such a group over time and collect clinical and biologic data, acknowledging the interaction of social and biologic factors.

The Georgia Lupus Registry (GLR) is 1 of 5 recently completed US Centers for Disease Control and Prevention (CDC)-funded population-based lupus registries designed to minimize many of these limitations.[12] In 2002, the CDC Arthritis Program supplied funding for the Georgia Department of Public Health (GA DPH) to conduct surveillance of SLE in 2 counties (Fulton and DeKalb) within the Atlanta metropolitan area with large African American populations. To avoid biased ascertainment and under-reporting as a result of recruiting large numbers of community patients, the GA DPH as a public health authority used its public health surveillance exemption to the Health Insurance Portability and Accountability Act (HIPPA) Privacy Rule (45 CFR, 164.512[b]) to obtain protected health information without written consent of the patient. The GA DPH contracted with Emory University as its designated agent to provide lupus expertise and manage the project. The primary sources of potential cases included hospitals, rheumatologists, nephrologists, and dermatologists in and around the catchment area. Administrative databases were queried for billing codes for lupus and related conditions. Secondary sources included laboratories, renal and cutaneous pathology, and queries in other population databases.

In addition to obtaining more accurate incidence and prevalence rates of SLE, the GLR has contributed to the understanding of disparities in SLE, including persistent and significant disparities in end-stage renal disease and mortality in African Americans compared with whites.[13,14] Relative to SLE, research on cutaneous lupus erythematosus has been sparse, with little known about the epidemiology in minority populations. The GLR produced minimum estimates of the incidence of chronic cutaneous lupus erythematosus (CCLE) and found similar disparities as seen for SLE.[15]

THE GEORGIANS ORGANIZED AGAINST LUPUS COHORT

The Georgians Organized Against Lupus (GOAL) Cohort is a population-based lupus cohort supported by the CDC of over 1000 individuals with lupu,s derived, in large part, from the GLR. Institutional review board approvals allowed patients identified in the GLR to be contacted directly and offered the opportunity to consent to be prospectively followed in the GOAL cohort, primarily through regular surveys utilizing patient-reported instruments and receiving other research opportunities, including the collection of related biospecimens. To minimize survival bias and to compensate for attrition, SLE patients with less than 5 years of disease are continually recruited from diverse hospitals and community rheumatologists and through Lupus Foundation of America, Georgia Chapter (LFA-GA) advertisements. CCLE participants have been enrolled from multiple sources, including the GLR, Grady Hospital, and Emory University dermatology clinics, referrals by community practices, and self-referrals facilitated by LFA-GA advertisements.

Consecutive annual sets of surveys have been administered to the GOAL cohort participants since 2012. All participants completed a self-report questionnaire to return via mail or completed via Internet or phone. In order to maximize participation, participants in the GOAL cohort who received care at Grady Memorial Hospital were recruited to complete the survey during their regularly scheduled clinic visit. Grady Hospital provides care for Atlanta's indigent and underinsured populations and has the only clinic dedicated to lupus care in the area. This was particularly helpful in capturing the most vulnerable patients, who are often socially disadvantaged and have difficulty completing surveys remotely.

Coordinating different questionnaire modalities and timelines for mailing and processing of returned surveys was accomplished through a sophisticated project management and database system developed for the GOAL cohort. The system generates paper-based or Internet-accessible surveys unique to each designated recipient. For clinic visits, the system generates Web-based case report forms. For participants who request it, phone interview-assisted surveys are given by the research coordinators using a standardized script and responses.

SOCIAL DETERMINANTS OF HEALTH IN THE GEORGIANS ORGANIZED AGAINST LUPUS COHORT

The GOAL research cohort is a rich and diverse repository of clinical, biological, sociodemographic, psychosocial, and health services data as well as biologic material (**Fig. 1**) that will improve the understanding of how various factors interact and may lead to interventions, on an individual as well as systems and societal level, that will help to mitigate the significant disparities that continue to exist in lupus.

Surveys have covered the domains of natural history, treatment, health care access and gaps, and disparities using validated instruments whenever possible (**Table 1**). Sociodemographic information was obtained, including employment, income,

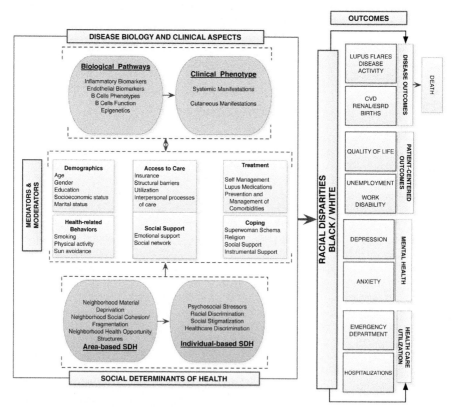

Fig. 1. Overall conceptual model of the GOAL cohort.

Table 1
Summary of measures and self-reported instruments

Major Domain	Category	Measure
Natural History	CVD	Incident and prevalent CVD
	ESRD	Incident ESRD
	Cancer	Incident cancer and cancer types
	Birth outcomes	Pregnancy risk factors, procedures, delivery method, maternal morbidity, newborn weight, abnormal conditions, birth defects, parent demographics
	Mortality	Death, cause(s) of death
	Violent death	Suicide and other violent deaths
	Disease severity	SLE disease activity, SLE organ damage, comorbidities, skin activity/chronicity
	Mental health	Depression, anxiety, anger, psychosocial illness impact, applied cognition, abilities, global health-mental, psychological distress
	Physical health	Physical function, bodily pain, pain interference, fatigue, sleep disturbance, global health-physical
	Social health	Social roles and activities, social isolation
	Skin-specific QoL	Emotions, functioning, symptoms, body image, photosensitivity
	Employment and work	Employment, disability, work productivity impairment
	Immune phenotypes and autoantibodies	Laboratory assays
	Inflammatory and endothelial markers	Laboratory assays
	Epigenetics	Laboratory assays
	Banked biospecimens	Laboratory assays
Treatment	Medications	Medications to treat lupus
	Opioids and pain medications	Prescription pain medication misuse, appeal of substance use, severity of substance use
	Self-management	Symptoms management self-efficacy, communication with physicians
	Alternative therapies	Complementary alternative medicine
	Treatment adherence	Medication management self-efficacy, treatment adherence
Health care	Access	Insurance, copayments
	Utilization	ED visits, hospitalizations
	Quality of care	Physician-patient interactions
		Quality of skin lupus care
		Health care experiences
		ESRD treatment-quality indicators

(continued on next page)

Major Domain	Category	Measure
Table 1 *(continued)*		
Disparities themes	Demographics	Age, sex, race, socioeconomic status, education
	Geographic and neighborhood factors	Material deprivation, social cohesion/fragmentation, neighborhood opportunity structures
	Social stressors and barriers	Discrimination, stigma (disease-related), neighborhood domains, financial strain, childhood trauma, self-perceived stress, experiences of prison
	Social support	Emotional, Informational, Instrumental
	Health-related behaviors	Smoking, drinking, physical activity, eating habits, sleep disorders, preventive care
		Coping mechanisms, social isolation, religion, spirituality

Abbreviations: CVD, cardiovascular disease; ED, emergency department; ESRD, end-stage renal disease; QoL, quality of life.

education, insurance, household composition, and relationship status. The surveys also included a detailed psychosocial battery, with measures of discrimination, other psychosocial stressors, and current mental health (eg, depression) and other social determinants that can potentially explain black/white disparities in this population.

Biospecimens from consenting GOAL participants have been collected and various immune and inflammatory assays have been analyzed to better understand the immune pathways across lupus phenotypes and the intersection between social determinants of health and biologic processes. DNA, RNA, and aliquots of serum and plasma are banked.

GOAL participants, as well as those in the GLR, have been matched with state and national databases, including the Georgia Hospital Discharge Database, National Death Index, Georgia Comprehensive Cancer Registry, US. Renal Data System, and Georgia Birth Records. Furthermore, all participants' addresses have been geocoded and linked to census information (tract and block group levels) and other area-based databases for socioeconomic, neighborhood, and other information.

CONTRIBUTIONS

These data provide powerful opportunities to explore the impact of social determinants in lupus and have yielded the following

- A self-management program benefits low-income African American women with SLE.[16]
- African Americans suffer higher rates of unemployment after lupus diagnosis.[17]
- Unfair treatment may contribute to worse disease outcomes among African American women with SLE.[18]
- Increasing frequency of racial discrimination was associated with greater SLE activity and damage in African American women.[19]
- Vicarious racism, or secondhand exposure to racism, was found to be associated with SLE activity after adjusting for socioeconomic and health-related covariates.[20]

- There is a high burden of cognitive symptoms and perceived stress in SLE.[21]
- Depressive symptoms are associated with low treatment adherence in African Americans with SLE.[22]
- There is a significant association between organ damage and depression in African American women, with social support being protective of depression.[23]
- The prevalence of depressive symptoms is high in a predominantly black cohort with primary CCLE.[24]
- Depression, which is highly prevalent in African American patients with SLE, may have a negative impact on physician-patient interactions.[25]
- African American women with SLE were more likely to experience a 12-month period of infertility, and at younger ages, but as likely as comparison women without SLE to have met their desired family size.[26]

SUMMARY

The GOAL research cohort was born out of the efforts of the GLR to create a population-based prospective cohort of validated SLE and cutaneous lupus patients, representing real-world lupus in an area where half of the population is African American or black. It is also an example of the power that can be harnessed by leveraging public health partnerships between federal, state, and academic institutions.

ACKNOWLEDGMENTS

The authors would like thank Charmayne Dunlop-Thomas, Associate Director of Research Projects, and Gaobin Bao, Senior Biostatistician, for their support of the GOAL research cohort, as well as Grady Memorial Hospital and all of the lupus patients.

Funding: Support for the GLR and GOAL cohort came under the following US Centers for Disease Control and Prevention cooperative agreements: DP08806, U01DP005119, U01DP006488.

DISCLOSURE

The authors have nothing to disclose.

REFERENCES

1. Brunsting LA. Disseminated (systemic) lupus erythematosus. Proc Staff Meet Mayo Clin 1952;27(22):410–2.
2. Harvey AM, Shulman LE, Tumulty PA, et al. Systemic lupus erythematosus: review of the literature and clinical analysis of 138 cases. Medicine (Baltimore) 1954; 33(4):291–437.
3. Siegel M, Holley HL, Lee SL. Epidemiologic studies on systemic lupus erythematosus. Comparative data for New York City and Jefferson County, Alabama, 1956-1965. Arthritis Rheum 1970;13(6):802–11.
4. Alarcon GS, McGwin G Jr, Uribe A, et al. Systemic lupus erythematosus in a multiethnic lupus cohort (LUMINA). XVII. Predictors of self-reported health-related quality of life early in the disease course. Arthritis Rheum 2004;51(3): 465–74.
5. Alarcon GS, McGwin G Jr, Roseman JM, et al. Systemic lupus erythematosus in three ethnic groups. XIX. Natural history of the accrual of the American College of Rheumatology criteria prior to the occurrence of criteria diagnosis. Arthritis Rheum 2004;51(4):609–15.

6. Costenbader KH, Desai A, Alarcon GS, et al. Trends in the incidence, demographics, and outcomes of end-stage renal disease due to lupus nephritis in the US from 1995 to 2006. Arthritis Rheum 2011;63(6):1681–8.

7. Hanly JG, Urowitz MB, Su L, et al. Seizure disorders in systemic lupus erythematosus results from an international, prospective, inception cohort study. Ann Rheum Dis 2012;71(9):1502–9.

8. Cooper GS, Treadwell EL, St Clair EW, et al. Sociodemographic associations with early disease damage in patients with systemic lupus erythematosus. Arthritis Rheum 2007;57(6):993–9.

9. Rhew EY, Manzi SM, Dyer AR, et al. Differences in subclinical cardiovascular disease between African American and Caucasian women with systemic lupus erythematosus. Transl Res 2009;153(2):51–9.

10. Pons-Estel GJ, Gonzalez LA, Zhang J, et al. Predictors of cardiovascular damage in patients with systemic lupus erythematosus: data from LUMINA (LXVIII), a multiethnic US cohort. Rheumatology 2009;48(7):817–22.

11. Alarcon G. The LUMINA study.. 2011. Available at: https://www.the-rheumatologist.org/article/the-lumina-study/. Accessed February 8, 2020.

12. Drenkard C, Lim SS. Update on lupus epidemiology: advancing health disparities research through the study of minority populations. Curr Opin Rheumatol 2019; 31(6):689–96.

13. Plantinga L, Lim SS, Patzer R, et al. Incidence of end-stage renal disease among newly diagnosed systemic lupus erythematosus patients: the Georgia Lupus Registry. Arthritis Care Res (Hoboken) 2016;68(3):357–65.

14. Lim SS, Helmick CG, Bao G, et al. Racial disparities in mortality associated with systemic lupus erythematosus - Fulton and DeKalb counties, Georgia, 2002-2016. MMWR Morb Mortal Wkly Rep 2019;68(18):419–22.

15. Drenkard C, Parker S, Aspey LD, et al. Racial disparities in the incidence of primary chronic cutaneous lupus erythematosus in the Southeastern US: the Georgia Lupus Registry. Arthritis Care Res (Hoboken) 2019;71(1):95–103.

16. Drenkard C, Dunlop-Thomas C, Easley K, et al. Benefits of a self-management program in low-income African-American women with systemic lupus erythematosus: results of a pilot test. Lupus 2012;21(14):1586–93.

17. Drenkard C, Bao G, Dennis G, et al. Burden of systemic lupus erythematosus on employment and work productivity: data from a large cohort in the southeastern United States. Arthritis Care Res (Hoboken) 2014;66(6):878–87.

18. Chae DH, Drenkard CM, Lewis TT, et al. Discrimination and cumulative disease damage among African American women with systemic lupus erythematosus. Am J Public Health 2015;105(10):2099–107.

19. Chae DH, Martz CD, Fuller-Rowell TE, et al. Racial discrimination, disease activity, and organ damage: the black women's experiences living with lupus (BeWELL) study. Am J Epidemiol 2019;188(8):1434–43.

20. Martz CD, Allen AM, Fuller-Rowell TE, et al. Vicarious racism stress and disease activity: the black women's experiences living with lupus (BeWELL) study. J Racial Ethn Health Disparities 2019;6(5):1044–51.

21. Plantinga L, Lim SS, Bowling CB, et al. Perceived stress and reported cognitive symptoms among Georgia patients with systemic lupus erythematosus. Lupus 2017;26(10):1064–71.

22. Heiman E, Lim SS, Bao G, et al. Depressive symptoms are associated with low treatment adherence in African American individuals with systemic lupus erythematosus. J Clin Rheumatol 2018;24(7):368–74.

23. Jordan J, Thompson NJ, Dunlop-Thomas C, et al. Relationships among organ damage, social support, and depression in African American women with systemic lupus erythematosus. Lupus 2019;28(2):253–60.

24. Hong J, Aspey L, Bao G, et al. Chronic cutaneous lupus erythematosus: depression burden and associated factors. Am J Clin Dermatol 2019;20(3):465–75.

25. Drenkard C, Bao G, Lewis TT, et al. Physician-patient interactions in African American patients with systemic lupus erythematosus: demographic characteristics and relationship with disease activity and depression. Semin Arthritis Rheum 2019;48(4):669–77.

26. Angley M, Lim SS, Spencer JB, Howards PP. Infertility among African American women with systemic lupus erythematosus compared to healthy women: A pilot study. Arthritis Care Res (Hoboken) 2019. Jul. https://doi.org/10.1002/acr.24022.

Use of Quality Measures to Identify Disparities in Health Care for Systemic Lupus Erythematosus

Shilpa Arora, MD[a], Jinoos Yazdany, MD, MPH[b],*

KEYWORDS

- Systemic lupus erythematosus (SLE) • Health care • Access to care
- Quality measures • Disparities

KEY POINTS

- Poor access to specialty care is a major factor driving poor outcomes in systemic lupus erythematosus (SLE). SLE patients who are racial/ethnic minorities, have low socioeconomic status, and with public insurance face difficulties in accessing specialty care.
- Application of quality measures has identified gaps in the care of SLE and disparities among different populations. Physician SLE volume and center experience are associated with better quality of care.
- Higher performance on quality measures correlates with improved outcomes in SLE.

INTRODUCTION

Health care in systemic lupus erythematosus (SLE) is complex owing to the heterogenous nature of the disease with diverse organ manifestations and unpredictable disease course. Substantial disparities exist in disease-related morbidity and mortality across genders, different age groups, ethnicities, socioeconomic backgrounds and geographic locations.[1-4] Measurement of health care quality can identify gaps in clinical care at an earlier stage, where interventions could be planned and implemented to improve outcomes and reduce disparities.

Funding: Dr. J. Yazdany is supported by the Alice Betts Chair in Arthritis Research and NIH/NIAMS K24 AR074534. The views expressed here are those of the authors and not necessarily NIH/NIAMS.
a Division of Rheumatology, Rush University Medical Center, 1611 West Harrison Street, Suite 510, Chicago, IL 60612, USA; b Division of Rheumatology, University of California, San Francisco, 1001 Potrero Avenue, Suite 3300, San Francisco, CA 94110, USA
* Corresponding author.
E-mail address: Jinoos.Yazdany@ucsf.edu

Rheum Dis Clin N Am 46 (2020) 623–638
https://doi.org/10.1016/j.rdc.2020.07.003
0889-857X/20/© 2020 Elsevier Inc. All rights reserved.

rheumatic.theclinics.com

The Institute of Medicine defines quality as "the degree to which health services for individuals and populations increase the likelihood of desired health outcomes and are consistent with current professional knowledge."[5] Donabedian's[6] framework of health care assessment lays out a systematic approach to measure quality of care and divides the components of care into structural, process and outcome measures with a linear relationship among them. Structural measures denote the structure of the settings in which care occurs. Examples of structural measures pertinent to SLE care are access to specialty care and insurance coverage. Process measures denote provider actions while delivering care. In SLE, process measures often reflect adherence to evidence-based clinical guidelines as well as communication with patients to ensure their understanding of recommended treatment. Lastly, outcome measures denote the effects of care on the health status of patients and populations. Important outcomes in SLE include disease activity, damage, quality of life, hospitalizations and mortality.

This article reviews key findings from the past decade of quality measurement in SLE, which has yielded important insights into where the health care system is working and where there are disparities and need for improvement. Two types of quality measures commonly used by researchers to understand quality of care in SLE are discussed: structural measures and process measures.

STRUCTURAL MEASURES AND ACCESS TO CARE

Access to rheumatology specialty care is uneven across geographic regions and insurance coverage and can have a profound impact on the treatment and outcomes of people with SLE.[7] Given the complexity of the disease, it is not surprising that studies have shown a strong relationship between physician experience in treating SLE and outcomes. For example, data from a large sample of hospitalized patients in California (n = 9989) showed that the risk of in-hospital mortality due to SLE was much lower at centers with more experience treating the disease for women, blacks, Hispanics, and those with public medical insurance or no insurance.[8] Compared with patients hospitalized at hospitals with less experience, patients at the hospitals with more experience were younger (mean age 43.7 years vs 51.1 years, respectively) and included fewer whites (39.5% vs 60.5%, respectively) and more patients were with public insurance (28.8% vs16.7%, respectively) or no medical insurance (7.1% vs 3.9%, respectively).[9] In another large population-based sample of SLE, patients who were hospitalized in New York or Pennsylvania (n = 15,509), physician SLE volume was shown to be inversely related to in-hospital mortality after adjusting for demographic characteristics, severity of illness, and hospital characteristics, signifying a volume outcome relationship in the care of SLE.[10] Data from the National Inpatient Sample (NIS) also has shown lower mortality in SLE patients at hospitals seeing more of these patients.[11]

Similar findings have emerged from research in the ambulatory setting. Comparison of SLE care between primary care physicians and specialists (rheumatologists, nephrologists, and dermatologists) in the Indian Health Service lupus registry comprising patients from the Alaska Native population showed that specialist diagnosis of SLE was associated with a higher likelihood of having SLE classification criteria documented, being tested for biomarkers of disease, and ever receiving treatment with hydroxychloroquine.[12] Another study has shown better quality of care in a subspecialty SLE clinic in comparison to general rheumatology clinic. No demographic differences were noted in the patient population between the 2 clinics, but patients seen in the subspecialty lupus clinic had longer duration of disease and met more numbers of the ACR criteria for lupus in comparison to general rheumatology clinic.[13] Moderate correlation also was shown between physician SLE volume and performance on quality measures in this study.[13] In addition, a recent study showed that quality of care for lupus nephritis was significantly higher at academic centers specializing in SLE than in community practices,[14] even after adjusting for sociodemographic and disease differences among patients. These findings support that specialty and subspecialty care are associated with higher-quality care in SLE.

Data from different studies suggest that low socioeconomic status, as proxied by insurance status or measured by self-reported income, is associated with lower quality of care. The incidence of end-stage renal disease (ESRD) due to lupus nephritis (LN) and its association with age at onset, type of insurance, and socioeconomic status were studied in a cross-sectional study using the US Renal Data System (n = 7971). Among patients with LN who developed ESRD, those with private medical insurance were older when they began ESRD treatment than those with Medicaid or no insurance. These findings suggest that progression to ESRD varies with medical insurance status, possibly because of differences in quality of care or access to care.[15] In a population-based ecological study, the incidence of ESRD due to SLE was found higher in zip codes with higher proportions of hospitalizations with Medicaid (P<.0001) and higher rates of hospitalizations for ambulatory care–sensitive conditions (thus avoidable hospitalizations), again suggesting that limited access to care may contribute to this complication of SLE.[16]

Racial/ethnic minorities and those with low socioeconomic status are less likely to receive timely specialty care. Using data from Medicare claims in the states of Colorado, Massachusetts, and Virginia, researchers found that African American women were less likely to receive referrals to rheumatology care for SLE.[17] Data from the Lupus Outcomes Study, which is a large, longitudinal cohort of physician-confirmed SLE, showed that Medicaid patients with SLE traveled longer distances to see an SLE physician, especially rheumatologists, and reported more visits to a general practitioner and emergency room for their SLE.[18] Assessment of the predictors of utilization of rheumatology subspecialty care in this cohort showed that older age, lower income, and male gender were associated with absence of rheumatology visits.[19] Data from the 2004 to 2007 interview wave of Lupus Outcomes Study participants showed that the number of physician visits for SLE varied by education level and neighborhood poverty.[20] Finally, among Medicaid recipients with lupus nephritis nationally, 1 in 8 patients were found to use the emergency room as a usual source of care, suggesting barriers to accessing appropriate ambulatory specialty care.[21]

Delays in initial SLE diagnosis and in receiving life-saving therapies, such as kidney transplantations, also have been documented. Low household income predicted delayed presentation (≥1 year) to a pediatric rheumatologist in childhood SLE in a study using a large registry of pediatric SLE patients (n = 598).[22] In another study, 64% of African Americans and 66% of Asians saw a specialist within 3 months of diagnosis, compared with 92% and 85% for whites and Hispanics, respectively. For those with a high-school education or less, 45% were referred to specialty care in the first 3 months compared with 81% of those with a higher level of education.[23] Predictors of kidney transplantation among children with ESRD due to lupus nephritis were studied using the US Renal Data System demonstrating significant inequalities. There were fewer kidney transplants among African American versus white patients (odds ratio [OR] 0.48; P<.001), Hispanic versus non-Hispanic patients (OR 0.63; P = .03), and those with Medicaid versus those with private insurance (OR 0.70; P = .03). Mortality among African American children was found almost double that among white children (OR 1.83; P<.001).[24] These studies build a compelling picture that access to care is uneven across racial/ethnic and socioeconomic groups with SLE in the United States and point to quality of care as 1 potential root cause of disparities in the disease.

Although no quality measures that examine structures of SLE care have been developed, the research, discussed previously, suggests that measures that monitor access to specialty care could help track and address health care disparities nationally. Moreover, given multiple studies showing that racial/ethnic minorities, those with public insurance and those with low socioeconomic status are at highest risk for poor access to care, such measures could provide data to target programs that aim to expand access. Examples of structural measures include the proportion of patients who are seen by a rheumatologist within 30 days of a suspected diagnosis of SLE or rheumatic disease or the proportion of patients with SLE who are seen by a specialist in the disease at least once per year. Beyond tracking measures, education programs should target primary care providers and insurance policy makers in areas with low performance on access measures, and telehealth programs should be explored to expand the reach of high-volume SLE centers.[25]

PROCESS QUALITY MEASURES

Process measures denote health care provider actions in delivering care for SLE. Assessment of process measures provides actionable targets for quality improvement given care of SLE patients often is fragmented among different specialists and primary care providers. Quality indicators assessing processes of care are defined as "retrospectively measurable elements of practice performance for which there is evidence or consensus that can be used to assess the quality of care provided and hence change it."[26] Different sets of quality indicators have been developed for use in SLE utilizing standardized development techniques, including systematic literature reviews, expert panels, and Delphi interviews. A brief description of these quality indicators along with the recommending study groups is summarized in **Table 1**.[27-32]

DISPARITIES IN PERFORMANCE ON QUALITY MEASURES

Application of quality measures in SLE across several studies provides insight into gaps in SLE care and factors accounting for the disparities in quality of care. Data from self-report of 13 of 20 SLE quality indicators[27] showed an overall performance rate of 65%, with variable performance on the individual measures[33] (**Table 2**). Factors associated with poor performance included younger age, fewer physician visits, and lack of health insurance. As discussed previously, higher SLE patient volume and care in subspecialty SLE clinics have been shown associated with better performance on quality indicators.[13] This study analyzed performance on 20 measures with significant differences in 8 of them between SLE clinics and general rheumatology clinics, suggesting the roles of physician expertise and SLE volume in providing better quality of care in SLE.

Studies of quality measures in lupus nephritis have shown similar results, with better performance at academic centers[14] and for those patients with more specialist visits.[21] Data from the Medicaid program across 47 US states and the District of Columbia showed that performance of quality measures for lupus nephritis was low especially for use of immunosuppressive agents (see **Table 2**).[21] In this cohort, younger individuals, African Americans, and Hispanics were more likely to receive immunosuppressive therapy and hydroxychloroquine; however, younger individuals

Table 1
Quality Indicators developed for systemic lupus erythematosus

Area Covered	Description
Diagnosis	Initial antibody testing, including ANA, dsDNA, and aPL abs,[27,29,30] and baseline labs, including CBC, creatinine, and UA[27,30]
Disease monitoring	Regular lab monitoring,[28,29,31] regular disease activity assessment through validated indices,[28,29] damage measurement,[29] and quality-of-life measurement[29]
Medications	Counseling prior to starting drugs[27,28,30]; screening for HBV, HCV, and TB prior to immunosuppressives[29]; regular labs for drug toxicity[27,29–31]; addition of steroid sparing agent[27,30,31]; addition of antimalarials[30]; ophthalmologic examination for hydroxychloroquine[28–31]; and screening for cataracts and glaucoma while on steroids[29,30]
Renal disease	Diagnosis of lupus nephritis with renal biopsy,[28,30] regular labs for monitoring,[27,28,30,31] treatment with immunosuppressives,[27,28,30] ACE inhibitor/ARB for proteinuria,[27,30,31] and BP control[27]
Prevention	Sun avoidance counseling,[27,28,30] influenza and pneumococcal vaccination,[27,29,30] and meningococcal and *Hemophilus influenzae* vaccination (in children)[30]
Bone health	Screening for osteoporosis,[27,30] calcium and vitamin D supplementation,[27,28,30,31] and treatment of osteoporosis[27,31]
Cardiovascular screening	Annual screening and treatment of risk factors, including diabetes, hypertension, smoking, and obesity[27,28,30,31]
Reproductive health	Counseling regarding teratogenicity of drugs and contraception use[27,32]; testing for SSA, SSB, and aPL abs[27,28,30,32]; and treatment of APS in pregnancy[27,32]
Miscellaneous	Treatment of APS,[28,31] record of comorbidities,[29] immunosuppressives for neuropsychiatric SLE,[30] and transfer of care to adult providers (in adolescents)[30]

Abbreviations: ACE, angiotensin converting enzyme inhibitor; ANA, antinuclear antibody; aPL abs, antiphospholipid antibodies; APS, antiphospholipid antibody syndrome; ARB, angiotensin receptor blocker; CBC, complete blood cell count; dsDNA, double-stranded deoxyribonucleic acid antibody; HBV, hepatitis B virus; HCV, hepatitis C virus; LAB, laboratory; SSA, Sjögren syndrome A; SSB, Sjögren syndrome B; TB, tuberculosis; UA, urinalysis.

were less likely to receive renal-protective antihypertensive medications. Researchers also found that a significant number of patients used the emergency department as their usual source of care, defined as having greater than 50% of their yearly health care encounters in that setting. Not surprisingly, this group was less likely to receive recommended care.

Preventive measures play a significant role in the care of SLE patients and have been found uneven across populations (see **Table 2**). Having a primary care provider increases the likelihood of getting preventive services, including measures related to bone health[34] and vaccinations against influenza and pneumococcal infections.[40] Younger women, nonwhite patients, and those with shorter disease duration get these recommendations less often.[35,41] Study of reproductive health measures, another important issue in SLE, has shown that rates of contraceptive counseling are low: 30% to 60% across studies (see **Table 2**). In a retrospective cohort from Denver (n = 122), younger age (R 0.93),

Table 2
Performance on quality measures across studies in systemic lupus erythematosus between 2010 and 2019

Study	Population	Method/Process Measure Studied	Sun Avoidance	Vaccinations	Bone Health	Medications	Lupus Nephritis	Reproductive Health	Others
Schmajuk et al,[35] 2010	n = 742 (127 eligible)	Self-report data on 3 measures of bone health	—	—	BMD screening (74%), calcium-vitamin D (58%), osteoporosis treatment (56%)	—	—	—	—
Yazdany et al,[40] 2010	n = 685	Self-report data on cancer screening and vaccinations	—	Influenza vaccine (59%), pneumococcal (60%)	—	—	—	—	Cervical cancer screening (70%), mammography (70%), colon cancer screening (62%)
Demas et al,[34] 2010	n = 200	Retrospective review of bone health measures and cardiovascular screening	—	—	BMD screening (59%), calcium-vitamin D (62%), osteoporosis treatment (86%)	—	—	—	CVD screening (5 risk factors) (3%), CVD screening (excluding smoking) (26%)

	n	Data source							
Yazdany et al,[36] 2011	n = 206	Self-report of contraceptive use and counseling	—	—	—	—	—	Contraceptive counseling (41%), consistent contraceptive use (78%)	—
Yazdany et al,[33] 2012	n = 814	Self-report data on 13 measures	Sun avoidance counseling (90%)	Influenza vaccine (80%), pneumococcal (69%)	Calcium-fitamin D (83%), BMD screening (56%), osteoporosis treatment (61%)	Counseling prior to initiation (68%), counseling on GC management plan (65%), Drug monitoring (69%), steroid-sparing agent (65%)	ACE inhibitor or ARB (49%), BP control (54%)	Contraception counseling (40%)	CVD screening (29%)
Yazdany et al,[21] 2014	n = 1711	Medicaid administrative data on 3 measures for lupus nephritis at 90 days after diagnosis	—	—	—	—	Immunosuppressives for LN (22%), ACE inhibitor or ARB (44%), antimalarials (36%)	—	—

(continued on next page)

Table 2
(continued)

Study	Population	Method/Process Measure Studied	Sun Avoidance	Vaccinations	Bone Health	Medications	Lupus Nephritis	Reproductive Health	Others
Quinzanos et al,[37] 2015	n = 122	Retrospective review of 2 measures on reproductive health	—	—	—	—	—	Antibody screening in pregnancy (SSA, SSB, and aPLs ab) (100%), contraception counseling (46%)	—

	n		Sun	Influenza	Calcium-vitamin D	Antimalarials	Lab	Antibody	CVD
Mina et al,[38] 2016	n = 483	Retrospective review of 26 measures in pediatric SLE patients across 7 centers	Sun avoidance (54%–99%)	Influenza vaccination (57%–100%)	Calcium-vitamin D (59%–100%), BMD screening (7%–90%)	Antimalarials (75%–100%), Steroid sparing agent (25%–100%), counseling about drugs (60%–100%), lab monitoring for drugs (86%–100%), eye screening (72%–96%)	Lab monitoring for lupus nephritis (50%–100%), kidney biopsy (50%–100%), immunosuppressives (83%–100%), ACE inhibitor or ARB (80%–100%)	Antibody screening in pregnancy (50%–100%)	CVD screening (0%–100%), transition of care (13%–100%), treatment of neuropsychiatric lupus (80%–100%)
Harris et al,[39] 2017	n = 75	Retrospective review of 7 measures in pediatric SLE	—	Influenza vaccine (76%), pneumococcal (32%), meningococcal (67%)	Vitamin D recommendation (84%), BMD screening (29%)	HCQ use (94%), eye screening (49%)	—	—	—

(continued on next page)

Table 2
(continued)

Study	Population	Method/Process Measure Studied	Sun Avoidance	Vaccinations	Bone Health	Medications	Lupus Nephritis	Reproductive Health	Others
Arora et al,[13] 2018	n = 150	Self-report and retrospective review on 20 measures	Sun avoidance (lupus clinic vs general rheumatology clinic; 99% vs 84%, respectively)[a]	Influenza vaccine (lupus clinic vs general rheumatology clinic; 98% vs 88%, respectively), pneumococcal (lupus clinic vs general rheumatology clinic; 85% vs 49%, respectively)[a]	Calcium-vitamin D (lupus clinic vs general rheumatology clinic; 78 vs 72%, respectively), BMD screening (lupus clinic vs general rheumatology clinic; 94% vs 54%, respectively),[a] osteoporosis treatment (100% in both clinics)	Counseling prior to drugs (lupus clinic vs general rheumatology clinic; 92% vs 81%, respectively),[a] steroid-sparing agent (lupus clinic vs general rheumatology clinic; 100% vs 82%, respectively)[a]	ACE inhibitor or ARB (lupus clinic vs general rheumatology clinic; 94% vs 58%, respectively),[a] BP control (lupus clinic vs general rheumatology clinic; 94% vs 100%, respectively), immunosuppressives (100% in both clinics)	Contraception counseling (lupus clinic vs general rheumatology clinic; 90% vs 65%, respectively)	CVD screening (lupus clinic vs general rheumatology clinic; 40% vs 15%, respectively),[a] aPLs ab testing (lupus clinic vs general rheumatology clinic; 72% vs 37%, respectively)[a]

| Aggarwal et al,[14] 2019 | n = 250 | Retrospective review of 8 measures for screening and treatment of lupus nephritis | — | — | — | — | Urine screening for nephritis (42%), kidney biopsy (67%), immunosuppressives (81%), BP control (78%) | — | Overall performance 85% at academic centers vs 60% at community centers[a] |

Abbreviations: ACE, angiotensin converting enzyme inhibitor; aPLs ab, antiphospholipid antibodies; ARB, angiotensin receptor blocker; BMD, bone mineral density; BP, blood pressure; CVD, cardiovascular disease; GC, glucocorticoid; HCQ, hydroxychloroquine; LAB, laboratory; LN, lupus nephritis; SSA, Sjogren's syndrome A; SSB, Sjogren's syndrome B.
[a] *P* value <.05.

and those who did not describe English as their primary language (OR 0.29) were more likely to have received counseling on drug teratogenicity.[37] A study of factors associated with contraception counseling in the Lupus Outcomes Study cohort showed that older age, white race, those with depressive symptoms, and higher SLE disease activity were less likely to get contraception counseling.[42]

Gaps in quality of care also have been demonstrated among children with SLE. Evaluation of quality indicators in a cohort of 75 childhood SLE patients showed especially low rates of bone mineral density evaluation (28.6%) and pneumococcal vaccination (31.7%).[39] In a large sample of childhood-onset SLE patients (n = 783), care differed markedly for several quality indicators addressing lupus nephritis, bone health, vaccinations, education on cardiovascular risk, and transition planning across different centers in the United states, Brazil, and India.[38] Access to kidney biopsies was found to be lower in Brazil than in the United States and, irrespective of the country, larger centers more often met the measures than smaller centers, reinforcing the volume-quality relationship seen in multiple US studies.

As evident from these study findings, process measures help identify gaps and disparities in care of SLE. SLE measures, however, are not deployed routinely in rheumatology clinics or federal programs. Using an online survey of 32 questions mailed to rheumatologists seeing adult SLE patients in academic settings, two-thirds of respondents reported being familiar with quality indicators in SLE, but only 18% reported using them in daily practice.[43] Most rheumatologists (81%) had a positive perception of the SLE quality indicators and agreed that their implementation could improve quality care in SLE, but they identified time as a barrier to implementation. Strategies to incorporate these measures in daily practice, such as alerts or checklists in electronic medical records, have been suggested. For instance, quality improvement methodology was applied in a study of 123 childhood SLE patients where a standardized previsit planning process to electronically pend orders for the needed screenings prior to a scheduled clinic visit was performed. This intervention increased the percentage of patients with completed screenings from 54% to 92% for annual vitamin D, 55% to 84% for annual lipid profiles, and 57% to 78% for bone density screening.[44] Such interventions may be beneficial in providing recommended care as well as saving time.

Importantly, longitudinal follow-up of SLE patients has demonstrated that higher performance on process quality measures improves outcomes over time. Higher performance on quality measures resulted in less accrual of damage in the Lupus Outcomes Study.[45] In another recent study, receiving higher-quality clinical care was associated with low disease activity, less progress in disease damage, and better quality of life at 2-year follow-up.[46] The impact of improving performance on SLE quality measures, however, in reducing disparities and other outcomes, such as costs, health care utilization, and overall mortality, still remains to be ascertained in longitudinal studies.

OUTCOME MEASURES

There remain significant challenges to developing outcome performance measures in SLE and none has been developed to date. Key SLE outcomes, such as accumulated organ damage, may take years to develop and, therefore, are perceived as not entirely within the immediate control of individual providers. In addition, risk adjustment of averaged patient outcomes within a clinic or health care system is daunting in a disease that can affect virtually any organ in the body and has dramatically different levels of severity in the population. Despite these challenges, research is beginning to lay a foundation for outcomes measurement in SLE, given that the ultimate goal of quality measurement is to improve patient outcomes.

Most work on outcome measures has examined inpatient quality of care. Studies assessing in-hospital mortality due to SLE have shown lower mortality at centers with more experience and higher physician SLE volume, as described previously. Hospital readmissions also are a potentially important outcome measure, given that SLE has the sixth highest readmission rate among all medical conditions in the United States.[47] One in 6 hospitalized patients with SLE is readmitted within 30 days of discharge.[48] Using hospital discharge databases from 5 geographically dispersed states, risk-adjusted hospital readmission rates have been shown significantly higher among at-risk populations, including racial/ethnic minorities and those with lower socioeconomic status.[48]

What about patients? What do they define as high quality? In formative work, researchers engaged individuals with SLE, a majority of whom were African American women from medically underserved communities, to discuss barriers to care and strategies for quality improvement.[49] Patients identified outcome measures that they think are most important, including measures of quality of life, functioning, mental health, and self-efficacy. More work is needed, but partnering with patients to further develop these priorities into quality measures will be important.

SUMMARY

Despite significant challenges posed by the complexity and relatively low prevalence of SLE and the multifaceted health care needed to treat it, the past decade of research has overcome some of these challenges to lay a framework for quality measurement and improvement. Process measures with specifications for a variety of data sources are available for use, and preliminary data suggest that better performance on process measures are associated with improved health outcomes in SLE. Outcome measures have been applied to assess quality during hospitalizations, and the results of these studies provide benchmarking information for researchers and health systems aiming to improve SLE care. Lastly, patients have identified several areas they think are critical for quality measurement.

Importantly, it has been learned that poor access to subspecialty care is a major threat to high-quality care in SLE and that providers with more experience treating SLE generally have better outcomes. Tracking and working to improve access to care, therefore, are major priorities for improving SLE care, as is ensuring that patients can benefit more broadly from the expertise of specialty centers. In addition, significant disparities in quality of care have been identified, with racial/ethnic minorities, low-income patients, and those with lower educational attainment and public insurance consistently having lower quality of care across studies. As recently stated by Sivashanker and Gandhi,[50] "there is no such thing as high-quality, safe care that is inequitable." Future work should focus on deployment of SLE quality measures across health systems and clinical data registries, and resulting data should be used to proactively address gaps in care and reduce health care disparities for the disease.

DISCLOSURES

No potential conflict of interests.

REFERENCES

1. Drenkard C, Lim SS. Update on lupus epidemiology: advancing health disparities research through the study of minority populations. Curr Opin Rheumatol 2019; 31(6):689–96.

2. Boodhoo KD, Liu S, Zuo X. Impact of sex disparities on the clinical manifestations in patients with systemic lupus erythematosus: A systematic review and meta-analysis. Medicine (Baltimore) 2016;95(29):e4272.

3. Falasinnu T, Chaichian Y, Palaniappan L, et al. Unraveling Race, Socioeconomic Factors, and Geographical Context in the Heterogeneity of Lupus Mortality in the United States. ACR Open Rheumatol 2019;1(3):164–72.

4. Singh RR, Yen EY. SLE mortality remains disproportionately high, despite improvements over the last decade. Lupus 2018;27(10):1577–81.

5. Institute of Medicine (US) Committee on quality of health care in America. Crossing the quality chasm: a New health system for the 21st century. Washington (DC): National Academies Press (US); 2001.

6. Donabedian A. The quality of care. How can it be assessed? JAMA 1988;260(12): 1743–8.

7. Schmajuk G, Tonner C, Yazdany J. Factors associated with access to rheumatologists for Medicare patients. Semin Arthritis Rheum 2016;45(4):511–8.

8. Ward MM. Hospital experience and mortality in patients with systemic lupus erythematosus: which patients benefit most from treatment at highly experienced hospitals? J Rheumatol 2002;29(6):1198–206.

9. Ward MM. Hospital experience and mortality in patients with systemic lupus erythematosus. Arthritis Rheum 1999;42(5):891-898.

10. Ward MM. Association between physician volume and in-hospital mortality in patients with systemic lupus erythematosus. Arthritis Rheum 2005;52(6):1646–54.

11. Tektonidou MG, Dasgupta A, Ward MM. Interhospital variation in mortality among patients with systemic lupus erythematosus and sepsis in the USA. Rheumatology (Oxford) 2019;58(10):1794–801.

12. McDougall JA, Helmick CG, Lim SS, et al. Differences in the diagnosis and management of systemic lupus erythematosus by primary care and specialist providers in the American Indian/Alaska Native population. Lupus 2018;27(7): 1169–76.

13. Arora S, Nika A, Trupin L, et al. Does systemic lupus erythematosus care provided in a lupus clinic result in higher quality of care than that provided in a general rheumatology clinic? Arthritis Care Res (Hoboken) 2018;70(12):1771–7.

14. Aggarwal I, Li J, Trupin L, et al. Quality of care for the screening, diagnosis, and management of lupus nephritis across multiple healthcare settings. Arthritis Care Res (Hoboken) 2019. https://doi.org/10.1002/acr.23915.

15. Ward MM. Medical insurance, socioeconomic status, and age of onset of end-stage renal disease in patients with lupus nephritis. J Rheumatol 2007;34(10): 2024–7.

16. Ward MM. Access to care and the incidence of end stage renal disease due to systemic lupus erythematosus. J Rheumatol 2010;37(6):1158–63.

17. Katz JN, Barrett J, Liang MH, et al. Utilization of rheumatology physician services by the elderly. Am J Med 1998;105(4):312–8.

18. Gillis JZ, Yazdany J, Trupin L, et al. Medicaid and access to care among persons with systemic lupus erythematosus. Arthritis Rheum 2007;57(4):601–7.

19. Yazdany J, Gillis JZ, Trupin L, et al. Association of socioeconomic and demographic factors with utilization of rheumatology subspecialty care in systemic lupus erythematosus. Arthritis Rheum 2007;57(4):593–600.

20. Tonner C, Trupin L, Yazdany J, et al. Role of community and individual characteristics in physician visits for persons with systemic lupus erythematosus. Arthritis Care Res (Hoboken) 2010;62(6):888–95.

21. Yazdany J, Feldman CH, Liu J, et al. Quality of care for incident lupus nephritis among Medicaid beneficiaries in the United States. Arthritis Care Res (Hoboken) 2014;66(4):617–24.

22. Rubinstein TB, Mowrey WB, Ilowite NT, et al, Childhood Arthritis and Rheumatology Research Alliance INVESTIGATORS. Delays to Care in Pediatric Lupus Patients: Data From the Childhood Arthritis and Rheumatology Research Alliance Legacy Registry. Arthritis Care Res (Hoboken) 2018;70(3):420–7.

23. Gaynon L, Katz PP, Dall'Era M, et al. Disparities in Access to Specialist Care at the Time of Diagnosis of Systemic Lupus Erythematosus [abstract]. Arthritis Rheumatol 2016;68(suppl 10). Available at: https://acrabstracts.org/abstract/disparities-in-access-to-specialist-care-at-the-time-of-diagnosis-of-systemic-lupus-erythematosus/. Accessed February 28, 2020.

24. Hiraki LT, Lu B, Alexander SR, et al. End-stage renal disease due to lupus nephritis among children in the US, 1995-2006. Arthritis Rheum 2011;63(7):1988–97.

25. Rezaian MM, Brent LH, Roshani S, et al. Rheumatology Care Using Telemedicine. Telemed J E Health 2019. https://doi.org/10.1089/tmj.2018.0256.

26. Campbell SM, Braspenning J, Hutchinson A, et al. Research methods used in developing and applying quality indicators in primary care. BMJ 2003;326(7393):816–9.

27. Yazdany J, Panopalis P, Gillis JZ, et al. Systemic Lupus Erythematosus Quality Indicators Project Expert Panels. A quality indicator set for systemic lupus erythematosus. Arthritis Rheum 2009;61(3):370–7.

28. Mosca M, Bombardieri S. Disease-specific quality indicators, guidelines, and outcome measures in systemic lupus erythematosus (SLE). Clin Exp Rheumatol 2007;25(6 Suppl 47):107–13.

29. Mosca M, Tani C, Aringer M, et al. Development of quality indicators to evaluate the monitoring of SLE patients in routine clinical practice. Autoimmun Rev 2011;10(7):383–8.

30. Hollander MC, Sage JM, Greenler AJ, et al. International consensus for provisions of quality-driven care in childhood-onset systemic lupus erythematosus. Arthritis Care Res (Hoboken) 2013;65(9):1416–23.

31. Yajima N, Tsujimoto Y, Fukuma S, et al. The development of quality indicators for systemic lupus erythematosus using electronic health data: A modified RAND appropriateness method. Mod Rheumatol 2019. https://doi.org/10.1080/14397595.2019.1621419.

32. Gillis JZ, Panopalis P, Schmajuk G, et al. Systematic review of the literature informing the systemic lupus erythematosus indicators project: reproductive health care quality indicators. Arthritis Care Res (Hoboken) 2011;63(1):17–30.

33. Yazdany J, Trupin L, Tonner C, et al. Quality of care in systemic lupus erythematosus: application of quality measures to understand gaps in care. J Gen Intern Med 2012;27(10):1326–33.

34. Demas KL, Keenan BT, Solomon DH, et al. Osteoporosis and cardiovascular disease care in systemic lupus erythematosus according to new quality indicators. Semin Arthritis Rheum 2010;40(3):193–200.

35. Schmajuk G, Yelin E, Chakravarty E, et al. Osteoporosis screening, prevention, and treatment in systemic lupus erythematosus: application of the systemic lupus erythematosus quality indicators. Arthritis Care Res (Hoboken) 2010;62(7):993–1001.

36. Yazdany J, Trupin L, Kaiser R, et al. Contraceptive counseling and use among women with systemic lupus erythematosus: a gap in health care quality? Arthritis Care Res (Hoboken) 2011;63(3):358–65.
37. Quinzanos I, Davis L, Keniston A, et al. Application and feasibility of systemic lupus erythematosus reproductive health care quality indicators at a public urban rheumatology clinic. Lupus 2015;24(2):203–9.
38. Mina R, Harris JG, Klein-Gitelman MS, et al. Initial Benchmarking of the Quality of Medical Care in Childhood-Onset Systemic Lupus Erythematosus. Arthritis Care Res (Hoboken) 2016;68(2):179–86.
39. Harris JG, Maletta KI, Kuhn EM, et al. Evaluation of quality indicators and disease damage in childhood-onset systemic lupus erythematosus patients. Clin Rheumatol 2017;36(2):351–9.
40. Yazdany J, Tonner C, Trupin L, et al. Provision of preventive health care in systemic lupus erythematosus: data from a large observational cohort study. Arthritis Res Ther 2010;12(3):R84.
41. Lawson EF, Trupin L, Yelin EH, et al. Reasons for failure to receive pneumococcal and influenza vaccinations among immunosuppressed patients with systemic lupus erythematosus. Semin Arthritis Rheum 2015;44(6):666–71.
42. Ferguson S, Trupin L, Yazdany J, et al. Who receives contraception counseling when starting new lupus medications? The potential roles of race, ethnicity, disease activity, and quality of communication. Lupus 2016;25(1):12–7.
43. Casey C, Chung CP, Crofford LJ, et al. Rheumatologists' perception of systemic lupus erythematosus quality indicators: significant interest and perceived barriers. Clin Rheumatol 2017;36(1):97–102.
44. Smitherman EA, Huang B, Furnier A, et al. Quality of care in childhood-onset systemic lupus erythematosus: Report of an intervention to improve cardiovascular and bone health screening. J Rheumatol 2019. https://doi.org/10.3899/jrheum.190295.
45. Yazdany J, Trupin L, Schmajuk G, et al. Quality of care in systemic lupus erythematosus: the association between process and outcome measures in the Lupus Outcomes Study. BMJ Qual Saf 2014;23(8):659–66.
46. Kernder A, Richter JG, Fischer-Betz R, et al. Quality of care predicts outcome in systemic lupus erythematosus: a cross-sectional analysis of a German long-term study (LuLa cohort). Lupus 2020;29(2):136–43.
47. Elixhauser A, Steiner C. Readmissions to U.S. Hospitals by Diagnosis, 2010: Statistical Brief #153. In: Healthcare Cost and Utilization Project (HCUP) Statistical Briefs. Rockville (MD): Agency for Healthcare Research and Quality (US); 2006.
48. Yazdany J, Marafino BJ, Dean ML, et al. Thirty-day hospital readmissions in systemic lupus erythematosus: predictors and hospital- and state-level variation. Arthritis Rheumatol 2014;66(10):2828–36.
49. Feldman CH, Bermas BL, Zibit M, et al. Designing an intervention for women with systemic lupus erythematosus from medically underserved areas to improve care: a qualitative study. Lupus 2013 Jan;22(1):52–62.
50. Sivashanker K, Gandhi TK. Advancing safety and equity together. N Engl J Med 2020;382(4):301–3.

Socioeconomic Status, Health Care, and Outcomes in Systemic Lupus Erythematosus

Kimberly DeQuattro, MD, MM[a],*, Edward Yelin, PhD[b]

KEYWORDS

• Poverty • Socioeconomic status • Systemic lupus erythematosus • Outcomes

KEY POINTS

- Individuals with systemic lupus erythematosus (SLE) who are poor face unmet financial, physical, and psychosocial needs that exacerbate worse long-term outcomes such as disease damage and quality of life.
- The most severe negative outcomes are among individuals with SLE who are poor and who live in areas of concentrated poverty.
- Among individuals with SLE, permanent exit from poverty is associated with less adverse outcomes compared with individuals who remain in poverty. Interventions that target the individual's poverty may result in better SLE outcomes.
- Research exposing health iniquities galvanizes health care providers to advocate for efforts to reduce disparities among the poor with SLE within medicine. Ending poverty among persons with SLE demands a greater societal commitment.

Research on the effect of lower socioeconomic status (SES) on health care and outcomes among persons with systemic lupus erythematosus (SLE) has been expanding over the last decade, joining the considerable work done on the effect of race and ethnicity in the onset, pathogenesis, and outcomes of this condition. There is overlap in the literature, primarily because the prevalence of SLE is higher and more severe among members of racial and ethnic minorities, including persons of African and Asian backgrounds as well as Hispanics from any racial background. However, much research has established that, once SLE onset—which may be driven by genetic factors such as continent of origin—has occurred, differences in health care and outcomes among persons with SLE are driven sharply by the SES of the individual.[1,2]

In this article, the authors review the evidence that compares the health care and outcomes of persons with SLE from lower socioeconomic backgrounds with that of

[a] Division of Rheumatology, University of California, San Francisco, Box 0500, San Francisco, CA 94143-0500, USA; [b] Division of Rheumatology and Philip R Lee Institute for Health Policy Studies, Box 0936, San Francisco, CA 94143-0936, USA
* Corresponding author.
E-mail address: Kimberly.dequattro@ucsf.edu

Rheum Dis Clin N Am 46 (2020) 639–649
https://doi.org/10.1016/j.rdc.2020.07.004
0889-857X/20/© 2020 Elsevier Inc. All rights reserved.
rheumatic.theclinics.com

the more affluent. Had this article been written a decade ago, the research reviewed would have been limited to a handful of studies showing the extent to which low SES was associated with access to and utilization of health care and outcomes. Recent studies have started to elucidate some of the mechanisms underlying these relationships, giving rise to some initial attempts to intervene to reduce the disparities by actions of health care providers and in community demonstration projects. This article provides an overview of what has been established in the authors' understanding of the relationship between SES and SLE and what is beginning to be done to overcome the effects of low SES.

THE FOUNDATION FOR UNDERSTANDING SOCIOECONOMIC STATUS AND SYSTEMIC LUPUS ERYTHEMATOSUS

The literature on SES and SLE builds on almost 2 centuries of work on SES, morbidity, and mortality. Beginning with the anecdotal observations of Frederick Engels on the geography of despair in Manchester, England[3] but then continuing with the systematic cumulation of data by John Snow on the prevalence of environmental threats to the longevity of the poor[4] and of Charles Booth on the confluence of personal and neighborhood adversity on a range of outcomes including, but not limited to death,[5] the Victorians began the quest to understand why low SES translates into illness and its sequelae. Although the Victorians were the first to make these observations, historical epidemiologists have established that the adverse health outcomes did not just arise in the industrial era. In one such study, Smith[6] observed that in the main cemetery in Glasgow Scotland in which all who died in that city were buried for close to a millennium, the length of life as documented on gravestones was highly correlated with the height of the gravestone, a proxy for wealth, for several centuries preceding the industrial revolution. Adverse outcomes of low SES have been the historical norm.

However, it is in the last several decades that we have begun to understand why. The foundational work again came from the United Kingdom. Marmot and colleagues[7,8] used data encompassing the entire British civil service to establish that with each step up the socioeconomic ladder, rates of morbidity of almost every condition and of mortality were lower. Because the British had established universal coverage half a century before this research was conducted, health care probably did not account for very much of the health disparities, although the authors acknowledge that there may be quality of care differences. In addition, they noted that the usual explanation other than health care is that persons of lower SES have more adverse health behaviors, for example, higher rates of smoking and heavy alcohol usage and greater levels of obesity; but this too did not account for the more adverse outcomes of those of lower SES.[9] If not due to health care and health behaviors, they hypothesized and then proved that the differences in health arose from the conditions of life in work and community, what we now call the social determinants of health.[10] These include poverty; the stresses associated with poverty, including, but not limited to, unemployment, underemployment, and poor working conditions; and the adverse conditions in the neighborhoods in which persons of low SES live.[11] This is the foundation for the studies of low SES and SLE to which we now turn.

POVERTY AND SYSTEMIC LUPUS ERYTHEMATOSUS

SLE disproportionately affects members of minority groups and the poor.[12] In US Medicaid data from 2000 to 2004, the prevalence of SLE was highest among the lowest quartile of area-level SES, independent of age, sex, or race/ethnicity (104.9 per 100,000, 95% confidence interval [CI] 99.8–110.3).[13] Although poverty is officially defined in countries such as the United States by a combination of income and household size, being poor is multidimensional and extends beyond lack of economic means alone. The concept of poverty also includes unmet social, physical, and political needs as important contributing factors to the impact of poverty on functioning in society. As a result of one or more of these factors, individuals with SLE of low SES have worse long-term disease outcomes[12] and poorer quality of life than those of higher SES.[14]

LONG-TERM OUTCOMES IN THE DISADVANTAGED WITH SYSTEMIC LUPUS ERYTHEMATOSUS

In addition to the impact of personal SES or frank poverty, there are effects of living in areas of concentrated poverty (areas in which a high proportion of the residents meet criteria for personal poverty) that may make the effect of personal poverty worse. In such areas, there may be limited access to basic human needs such as food, health, and medical care. There are potential adverse effects of toxic environmental exposures ranging from traffic to factories, prejudice and crime. Further, living in such areas may result in discrimination in housing, making it difficult to move to safer areas even when money is available to do so. With negative effects of living in areas of concentrated poverty, those with SLE living under such conditions may experience stigmatization and further marginalization. Residents of these areas report higher levels of perceived stress. The marginalization and fear associated with crime in the neighborhood may lead residents to spend more time within their households, curtailing their ability to take advantage of the social networks they have and limiting the reach of their network.[15]

Personal poverty alone but especially in combination with living in areas of concentrated poverty may result in higher levels of organ damage. Greater organ damage portends increased long-term disability and mortality in SLE. It is estimated that those who are poor with SLE live 14 fewer years than their nonpoor counterparts.[16] Recent studies suggest an intricate relationship among poverty, damage, and mortality.[17] Low income is directly associated with SLE damage in proportion to the degree of economic deprivation. With each lower level of income, the degree of organ damage increases. Similarly, there is a dose effect of living in poverty such that those who are persistently poor accrue more organ damage than those who are intermittently poor.[15]

Living in a state of concentrated poverty exaggerates personal poverty in those with SLE. Individuals living in areas of concentrated poverty experience higher levels of damage than those who are poor but not living in areas of concentrated poverty and the nonpoor regardless of where they live. Although many individual and community characteristics beyond poverty affect the level of organ damage, even after taking a wide array of those factors into account, the effect of personal and community poverty on organ damage remains profound. Examples of factors include degree of cognitive impairment; depression; health behaviors such as smoking, exercise, and diet; and the extent and quality of health care. The strong effect of living in concentrated poverty on SLE damage can be mitigated by exiting poverty. Exiting poverty permanently puts one on a more benign course of organ damage so that within a year or so, those who have left poverty have a disease course much like those who were never poor,[18] which suggests that the effects of being poor are mutable and not inherent in the people who are poor but rather by the fact of their current low incomes. It also suggests that programs to alleviate poverty and blunt the effects of living in areas of concentrated poverty may help persons with SLE avoid higher levels of disease damage.

BARRIERS TO IMPROVING LONG-TERM OUTCOMES AMONG POOR WITH SYSTEMIC LUPUS ERYTHEMATOSUS: DIRECT, INDIRECT, AND INTANGIBLE COSTS

The chronic multisystem course of SLE, often with cycles of flares and quiescence, yields high patient costs. Direct SLE-associated expenditures include hospitalizations, outpatient follow-up, medications, and transportation. Indirect costs due to disability from SLE sequelae include losses in productivity and employment. A litany of intangible humanistic costs affect quality of life in SLE. Each of these 3 types of costs is exacerbated in poverty with long-term adverse outcomes in SLE.

Direct Costs: Systemic Lupus Erythematosus is Expensive for the Poor

Cost for medical care, including medications, is high in SLE. Estimates for mean annual direct cost for US patients with SLE ranged from $13,735 to 20,926 (USD 2009), with costs for SLE nephritis exceeding 2 to 3 times those estimates. Expenses are distributed among inpatient (14%–50%), outpatient (24%–56%), and medication costs (19%–30%).[19] Although they fluctuate, costs persist over time, which can especially burden the poor and uninsured. Even in a universal health care setting in Canada, there were higher direct medical costs over time in those with a lower SES.[14] The reason for this disparity despite universal health care is unclear. One possibility is that those who are poor incur greater hospital costs, given they have more severe disease and often compromised access to outpatient care.

Access to care is a known challenge in SLE.[20] In the United States, despite Medicaid services, those with income levels less than $40,000 have fewer visits to a rheumatologist and travel a greater distance to access their care teams.[21,22] Poor patients living with SLE experience greater avoidable hospitalizations. Avoidable hospitalizations are preventable by prompt and appropriate treatments. In addition, a proportion of the direct cost for poor patients with SLE care may be associated with hospital readmissions. Based on administrative data, there are more frequent 30-day hospital readmissions among those who already tend to have lower SES and live in poverty: those of the youngest age, nonwhite racial/ethnic (African American and Hispanic), and publicly insured groups.[12,23]

Processes of care, such as care quality, are factors in the direct cost equation. Those who live in poverty report lower ratings of health plan interactions, such as health care utilization and technical quality of care, and experience worse patient-reported damage.[24] It is possible that in the setting of lesser quality of available care, some patients will need repeat visits to emergency departments or hospitals, which associate with more frequent admissions and utilization, driving up costs.

These examples suggest that patients with lower SES experience health inequities at a health care systems and delivery level.[25] Because those who experience poverty do not necessarily report inadequate patient-provider communication, there may be potential protective value in strengthening trust between a patient and their care team. There is ample evidence to support improvements in health care delivery for positive engagement of the poor toward improved long-term outcomes in SLE.

Indirect Costs: Education and Employment Are Disrupted

SLE affects patients during key years of productivity, when disruption of education and career are likely. High rates of career changes, interruptions, or complete work loss is a global problem among patients with SLE, with 20% to 50% reporting work loss after initial diagnosis.[26–28] The estimated annual loss in indirect costs for patients with SLE in the United States was $8659 (USD 2004).[29] In a multiethnic study, poverty and severe disease were among factors that predicted self-reported disability.[30] Patients who are already poor are less likely to be working at the time of diagnosis.[27] Unemployed individuals with SLE tend to be either receiving Medicare/Medicaid or are uninsured.[31] Because exit from poverty implies the ability to earn a living wage, discerning how to improve life for those with SLE of lower SES via job security is critical.

Studies among adults with childhood-onset SLE (cSLE) demonstrate that although patients often complete their education, they do not maintain consistent employment in adulthood.[32] In addition, individuals with cSLE who grow up in an environment with low household income frequently report disability.[33] Patterns of low SES and high disability increase vulnerability for adults with cSLE and identify them as a special subgroup that need resources that point them toward career success.

High and recurrent direct costs of care have dire consequences for those living in poverty SLE. Worse disability increases risks of health care loss, especially for those not eligible for Social Security Disability Insurance (SSDI) because SSDI beneficiaries are entitled to Medicare benefits 2 years after being approved for SSDI benefits. Loss of health insurance and means to support all but basic needs may lead to inability to make regularly scheduled appointments or obtain medications. These individuals become higher utilizers of emergent care services at risk of greater direct costs.[34] The extreme challenge of living in poverty with SLE extends past the individual level to the community and beyond: patients may rely on family or friends to pay for or provide housing and/or may need assistance from government-provided Supplemental Security Income and Supplemental Nutrition Assistance Program (formerly referred to as food stamps) to survive.[35] Career rehabilitation resources should be available to individuals with SLE living in poverty.

Humanistic Costs: Depression and Stress Affect Quality of Life

Direct and indirect costs of SLE do not operate in isolation. The humanistic costs of SLE—quality of life, mental health, social, and societal support—affect each other and play a role in indirect and direct costs.[36] Intangible costs are magnified by poverty: worse quality of life is common among those with SLE who have a low SES[37] and is associated with SLE-related disability as mediated by depression and perceived stress.[38]

Major depression or depressive symptoms are estimated to occur in 24% and 39% of patients with SLE, respectively,[39] with a negative impact on organ-related damage and quality of life.[40] Although poverty is not always one of the primary factors in this relationship,[41] it can play a role. For example, both individual and neighborhood SES are associated with greater depression.[18] One distinction between prevalent and incident depression is that individuals with a lower SES are more likely to have a high burden of depression at baseline. In addition, women who perceive high financial strain over time are at risk for new onset depression.[14] The degree to which depression affects poor individuals with SLE merits a dedicated focus for health improvement.

Stress has long been thought to drive disease onset and flares in SLE.[42] Recent data support an increased risk of incident SLE among those with a history of trauma in childhood or adulthood.[43,44] Exposure to adverse childhood experiences (ACEs) such as abuse, neglect, and household challenges before age 18 years can negatively affect adult health in a dose-response manner.[45] Individuals with a higher burden of ACEs reported worse SLE disease activity, damage, depression, and health status.[46] Depression and posttraumatic stress disorder play a significant role in coping with stressors in SLE.[47] Those living in poverty with SLE are vulnerable to early, chronic stress. A focus on the types as well as the timing, duration, and concentration of stress in those with SLE who live in poverty will help to better understand humanistic costs via stress and poverty. This knowledge can guide targeted programs to promote resilience among those with low SES.

MODIFIABLE FACTORS IN POVERTY AND SYSTEMIC LUPUS ERYTHEMATOSUS

The past 2 decades make clear the argument that poverty negatively influences important objective and subjective health outcomes in SLE such as organ damage and quality of life. Health care systems and teams should target modifiable factors both internal and external to health care to facilitate an improved life course in low income patients with SLE.

Interventions Internal to Health Care

Improve access to systemic lupus erythematosus care
Comprehensive medical homes for rheumatologic conditions and especially for SLE replete with mental health services, physical therapy, social work, and primary care could remove some barriers to access for patients who are living in poverty. Mental health care is of utmost import for this population, and greater efforts to secure timely visits for depression and other conditions are justified. Same day clinic visits for rheumatology and other specialists such as nephrology can minimize costs. Because individuals with SLE of lower SES travel greater distances from their rheumatology care,[22] mobile clinics, home visits, or rideshares could remove geographic barriers between patients and their care teams. A rideshare intervention for Medicaid patients in 2 urban, low-income academic primary care clinics failed to demonstrate improved no-show rates.[48] Therefore, needs assessments specific to low-income patients with SLE and transportation concerns could identify factors impeding travel to visits, such as work obligations. Telemedicine visits at home or at community centers could permit patients with responsibilities such as childcare to attend visits. Telehealth is well suited to effect change for poor patients with SLE. Finally, patient navigators with specialized training in assisting those with low income could help SLE patients as they move through the health care system.

Improve technical quality of care
The poor have more severe disease and are high utilizers of primary, community and academic care services. Technical quality of care relies on dissemination and use of the most up-to-date SLE and preventive care guidelines. Low-income patients may not interact principally with a rheumatologist during their visits for their SLE.[21] There is a need for leading rheumatology bodies to develop SLE medical education modules and toolkits to address standards of care for those living in poverty and to provide current information for trainees, emergency physicians, primary care physicians, and hospitalists. For example, a partnership between the American College of Rheumatology and the Lupus Initiative has made important strides in awareness about disparities among minorities with SLE by creating education tools for community practitioners.[49] Additional work can expand to address poverty specifically and promote these efforts to rheumatologists nationwide for dissemination among community stakeholders.

Improve interpersonal quality of care
In some instances, the poor have reflected positively on the patient-provider dyad.[24] In contrast, some patients have negative experiences with care teams. Negative

perceptions can be heightened when low-income patients are depressed and have high disease activity.[50] Because perceptions can change behaviors, materials sensitive to SES should be used to educate care teams about how to build positive relationships with individuals living with poverty and SLE. An important tool is shared decision-making, which strengthens the patient-provider bond by promoting self-efficacy around a common goal of the SLE care plan.

Interventions External to Health Care

Provide educational/vocational resources
Because education and navigating a job search are skills relevant to employment and, ideally, release from poverty, services that assist with educational and vocational programs are invaluable. An adolescent employment readiness center at Children's National Hospital facilitated academic and career counseling to teenagers.[51] Because of profound disruption of education and employment for this population, strategies on how to minimize gaps in work and enable those with SLE to continue to be gainfully employed should be rigorously explored and tested.

Promote independence with social health
Peer support programs have long been used in other diseases to build community and understanding of symptoms and treatment goals. Several academic-community partnerships curated and tested SLE awareness programs for Latino[52] and African American[53] communities. In addition, a peer-mentor–based project designed to build independence as well as improve outcomes and quality of life for African American women with SLE is underway.[54] Tailoring programs to specifically address the needs of those who are living in poverty is essential.

Champion resilience
The multifactorial stresses of living in poverty require individual, community, and systemic action to improve disease outcomes and quality of life. At the individual level, successful programs will help patients manage stress and support resilience to improve negative effects on quality of life. One patient-centered pilot, the Chronic Disease Self-Management Program, positively affected self-management behaviors and decreased health care utilization among low-income patients with SLE.[55] Systemic shifts to develop and use trauma-informed care modules are also underway.[56] Stress and ACEs differentiate the life course and heighten risk for poor outcomes in SLE. Strategies on how to prevent or repair effects of ACEs are needed, particularly in the context of poverty. In addition, disadvantaged communities need representation in research: conscious efforts must be made to provide infrastructure to include these groups so that there can be accurate exploration of how poverty, mental health, and stress can be mitigated in patients with SLE.

SUMMARY

In the last several decades, a series of studies have moved from recognizing that individuals with SLE living in poverty have worse outcomes to beginning to evaluate the mechanisms of why those patterns exist. We can expect the next decade to yield a greater focus on the mechanisms described with additional insight into how poverty affects coping with SLE. Deeper understanding of how poverty affects direct, indirect, and humanistic costs can inform which modifiable factors might be successful targets for interventions to minimize disparities in this vulnerable group of patients. Motivation to eliminate poverty and minimize adverse stressors should come from within and outside of the health care sphere.

DISCLOSURE

The authors have nothing to disclose.

REFERENCES

1. Alarcon GS. Lessons from LUMINA: a multiethnic US cohort. Lupus 2008;17(11): 971–6.
2. Demas KL, Costenbader KH. Disparities in lupus care and outcomes. Curr Opin Rheumatol 2009;21(2):102–9.
3. Engels F, Kiernan V. The conditions of the working class in England. 15th edition. Middlesex (England): Penguin; 1987.
4. Cameron D, Jones I. John Snow, the broad street pump and modern epidemiology. Int J Epidemiol 1983;12:393–6.
5. Booth C. Life and labour of the people in London: first results of an inquiry based on the 1891 census. J R Stat Soc 1893;56:557–93.
6. Smith GD, Carroll D, Rankin S, et al. Socioeconomic differentials in mortality: evidence from Glasgow graveyards. Br Med J 1992;305(6868):1554–7.
7. Marmot MG, Stansfeld S, Patel C, et al. Health inequalities among British civil servants: the Whitehall II study. Lancet 1991;337(8754):1387–93.
8. Marmot MG, Bosma H, Hemingway H, et al. Contribution of job control and other risk factors to social variations in coronary heart disease incidence. Lancet 2013; 9:69–74.
9. Marmot M. Social determinants of health. Clin Med (Northfield) 2005;5:244–8.
10. Raphael D. Social determinants of health: an overview of key issues and themes. In: Raphael D, editor. Social determinants of health. Toronto: Canadian Scholars' Press; 2009. p. 2–19.
11. Glymour M, Avendano M, Kawachi I. Socioeconomic status and health. In: Berkman L, Kawachi I, Glymour M, editors. Social epidemiology. New York: Oxford University Press; 2014. p. 17–62.
12. Peschken CA, Katz SJ, Silverman E, et al. The 1000 Canadian faces of lupus: Determinants of disease outcome in a large multiethnic cohort. J Rheumatol 2009; 36(6):1200–8.
13. Feldman CH, Hiraki LT, Liu J, et al. Epidemiology and sociodemographics of systemic lupus erythematosus and lupus nephritis among US adults with Medicaid coverage, 2000-2004. Arthritis Rheum 2013;65(3):753–63.
14. Mccormick N, Trupin L, Yelin EH, et al. Socioeconomic Predictors of Incident Depression in Systemic Lupus Erythematosus. Arthritis Care Res 2018;70(1): 104–13.
15. Yelin E, Trupin L, Yazdany J. A Prospective study of the impact of current poverty, history of poverty, and exiting poverty on accumulation of disease damage in systemic lupus erythematosus. Arthritis Rheumatol 2017;69(8):1612–22.
16. Yelin E, Yazdany J, Trupin L. Relationship Between Poverty and Mortality in Systemic Lupus Erythematosus. Arthritis Care Res 2018;70(7):1101–6.
17. Meacock R, Dale N, Harrison MJ. The humanistic and economic burden of systemic lupus erythematosus: A systematic review. Pharmacoeconomics 2013; 31(1):49–61.
18. Trupin L, Tonner MC, Yazdany J, et al. The role of neighborhood and individual socioeconomic status in outcomes of systemic lupus erythematosus. J Rheumatol 2008;35(9):1782–8.

19. Slawsky KA, Fernandes AW, Fusfeld L, et al. A structured literature review of the direct costs of adult systemic lupus erythematosus in the US. Arthritis Care Res 2011;63(9):1224–32.
20. Lawson EF, Yazdany J. Healthcare quality in systemic lupus erythematosus: Using Donabedian's conceptual framework to understand what we know. Int J Clin Rheumtol 2012;7:95–107.
21. Yazdany J, Gillis JZ, Trupin L, et al. Association of socioeconomic and demographic factors with utilization of rheumatology subspecialty care in systemic lupus erythematosus. Arthritis Care Res 2007;57(4):593–600.
22. Gillis JZ, Yazdany J, Trupin L, et al. Medicaid and access to care among persons with systemic lupus erythematosus. Arthritis Care Res 2007;57(4):601–7.
23. Yazdany J, Marafino BJ, Dean ML, et al. Thirty-day hospital readmissions in systemic lupus erythematosus: Predictors and hospital- and state-level variation. Arthritis Rheumatol 2014;66(10):2828–36.
24. Yelin E, Yazdany J, Tonner C, et al. Interactions between patients, providers, and health systems and technical quality of care. Arthritis Care Res 2015;67(3): 417–24.
25. Ward MM. Avoidable hospitalizations in patients with systemic lupus erythematosus. Arthritis Care Res 2008;59(2):162–8.
26. Mak A. The economic burden of systemic lupus erythematosus in Asia: the current state. Lupus 2010;19:1442–6.
27. Yelin E, Trupin L, Katz P, et al. Work dynamics among persons with systemic lupus erythematosus. Arthritis Care Res 2007;57(1):56–63.
28. Gordon C, Isenberg D, Lerstrøm K, et al. The substantial burden of systemic lupus erythematosus on the productivity and careers of patients: A European patient-driven online survey. Rheumatol (United Kingdom) 2013;52(12): 2292–301.
29. Panopalis P, Yazdany J, Gillis JZ, et al. Health care costs and costs associated with changes in work productivity among persons with systemic lupus erythematosus. Arthritis Care Res 2008;59(12):1788–95.
30. Bertoli AM, Fernández M, Alarcón GS, et al. Systemic lupus erythematosus in a multiethnic US cohort LUMINA (XLI): Factors predictive of self-reported work disability. Ann Rheum Dis 2007;66(1):12–7.
31. Drenkard C, Bao G, Dennis G, et al. Burden of systemic lupus erythematosus on employment and work productivity: Data from a large cohort in the southeastern United States. Arthritis Care Res 2014;66(6):878–87.
32. Lawson EF, Hersh AO, Trupin L, et al. Educational and vocational outcomes of adults with childhood- and adult-onset systemic lupus erythematosus: Nine years of followup. Arthritis Care Res 2014;66(5):717–24.
33. Hersh AO, Case SM, Son MB. Predictors of disability in a childhood-onset systemic lupus erythematosus cohort: results from the CARRA Legacy Registry. Lupus 2018;27(3):494–500.
34. Panopalis P, Gillis JZ, Yazdany J, et al. Frequent use of the emergency department among persons with systemic lupus erythematosus. Arthritis Care Res 2010;62(3):401–8.
35. Yelin E, Trupin L, Bunde J, et al. Poverty, neighborhoods, persistent stress, and systemic lupus erythematosus outcomes: a qualitative study of the patients' perspective. Arthritis Care Res 2019;71(3):398–405.
36. Elera-Fitzcarrald C, Fuentes A, González LA, et al. Factors affecting quality of life in patients with systemic lupus erythematosus: important considerations and potential interventions. Expert Rev Clin Immunol 2018;14(11):915–31.

37. Carter EE, Barr SG, Clarke AE. The global burden of SLE: Prevalence, health disparities and socioeconomic impact. Nat Rev Rheumatol 2016;12(10):605–20.

38. Sumner LA, Olmstead R, Azizoddin DR, et al. The contributions of socioeconomic status, perceived stress, and depression to disability in adults with systemic lupus erythematosus. Disabil Rehabil 2019;1–6. https://doi.org/10.1080/09638288.2018.1522550.

39. Zhang L, Fu T, Yin R, et al. Prevalence of depression and anxiety in systemic lupus erythematosus: A systematic review and meta-analysis. BMC Psychiatry 2017;17(1). https://doi.org/10.1186/s12888-017-1234-1.

40. Jordan J, Thompson NJ, Dunlop-Thomas C, et al. Relationships among organ damage, social support, and depression in African American women with systemic lupus erythematosus. Lupus 2019;28(2):253–60.

41. Knight AM, Trupin L, Katz P, et al. Depression risk in young adults with juvenile- and adult-onset lupus: twelve years of followup. Arthritis Care Res 2018;70(3):475–80.

42. Wallace DJ. The role of stress and trauma in rheumatoid arthritis and systemic lupus erythematosus. Semin Arthritis Rheum 1987;16(3):153–7.

43. Roberts AL, Malspeis S, Kubzansky LD, et al. Association of trauma and posttraumatic stress disorder with incident systemic lupus erythematosus in a longitudinal cohort of women. Arthritis Rheumatol 2017;69(11):2162–9.

44. Feldman CH, Malspeis S, Leatherwood C, et al. Association of childhood abuse with incident systemic lupus erythematosus in adulthood in a longitudinal cohort of women. J Rheumatol 2019;46(12):1589–96.

45. Anda RF, Felitti VJ, Bremner JD, et al. The enduring effects of abuse and related adverse experiences in childhood: A convergence of evidence from neurobiology and epidemiology. Eur Arch Psychiatry Clin Neurosci 2006;256(3):174–86.

46. DeQuattro K, Trupin L, Li J, et al. Relationships between adverse childhood experiences and health status in systemic lupus erythematosus. Arthritis Care Res (Hoboken) 2019. https://doi.org/10.1002/acr.23878.

47. Feldman CH, Costenbader KH, Solomon DH, et al. Area-level predictors of medication nonadherence among US medicaid beneficiaries with lupus: a multilevel study. Arthritis Care Res 2019;71(7):903–13.

48. Chaiyachati KH, Hubbard RA, Yeager A, et al. Association of rideshare-based transportation services and missed primary care appointments: A clinical trial. JAMA Intern Med 2018;178(3):383–9.

49. The Lupus Initiative. Availble at: https://thelupusinitiative.org/. Accessed May 20, 2020.

50. Drenkard C, Bao G, Lewis TT, et al. Physician–patient interactions in African American patients with systemic lupus erythematosus: Demographic characteristics and relationship with disease activity and depression. Semin Arthritis Rheum 2019;48(4):669–77.

51. Miller ML, White PH. The challenge of caring for indigent children with rheumatologic diseases. Am J Dis Child 1991;145(5):554–8.

52. Mancera-Cuevas K, Canessa P, Chmiel JS, et al. Addressing lupus health disparities: the MONARCAS community and academic collaborative program. Health Equity 2018;2(1):145–51.

53. Phillip CR, Mancera-Cuevas K, Leatherwood C, et al. Implementation and dissemination of an African American popular opinion model to improve lupus awareness: an academic–community partnership. Lupus 2019;28(12):1441–51.

54. Williams EM, Egede L, Oates JC, et al. Peer approaches to self-management (PALS): Comparing a peer mentoring approach for disease self-management

in African American women with lupus with a social support control: Study protocol for a randomized controlled trial. Trials 2019;20(1):1–13.

55. Drenkard C, Dunlop-Thomas C, Easley K, et al. Benefits of a self-management program in low-income African-American women with systemic lupus erythematosus: Results of a pilot test. Lupus 2012;21(14):1586–93.

56. Oral R, Ramirez M, Coohey C, et al. Adverse childhood experiences and trauma informed care: The future of health care. Pediatr Res 2016;79(1–2):227–33.

II. Understanding Disease and Population-Specific Rheumatic Disease Disparities

Understanding the Disproportionate Burden of Rheumatic Diseases in Indigenous North American Populations

Elizabeth D. Ferucci, MD, MPH

KEYWORDS

- Indigenous • Rheumatic disease • Autoimmune disease • Epidemiology
- Health disparities

KEY POINTS

- There is an excess burden of many rheumatic diseases in Indigenous North American populations in the United States and Canada.
- Understanding the epidemiology of rheumatic diseases in indigenous populations is important for physicians, health care organizations, and the communities affected by the high burden of disease. This information can ensure the necessary allocation of health care resources as well as education of health care providers and community members.
- Risk factors associated with high rates of rheumatic disease in indigenous populations have not been fully elucidated, but likely include a combination of multiple genetic and environmental factors.

INTRODUCTION

Studies have found a high incidence and prevalence of several rheumatic diseases in indigenous North American (INA) populations in the United States and Canada (**Table 1**). In the 1980s and 1990s, studies focused on high rates of rheumatoid arthritis (RA) in INA populations and the associated HLA alleles,[1] as well as high rates of spondyloarthritis in association with HLA B27 positivity.[2] Recent studies have expanded on the increased risk of RA in relatives and those with preclinical autoantibodies.[3] In addition, the Centers for Disease Control and Prevention (CDC)-funded lupus registries recently evaluated the epidemiology of systemic lupus erythematosus (SLE) across all racial and ethnic categories in the United States and documented the highest prevalence of SLE in American Indian/Alaska Native (AI/AN) women.[4]

Division of Community Health Services, Department of Clinical and Research Services, Alaska Native Tribal Health Consortium, 3900 Ambassador Drive, Suite 201, Anchorage, AK 99508, USA
E-mail address: edferucci@anthc.org

Rheum Dis Clin N Am 46 (2020) 651–660
https://doi.org/10.1016/j.rdc.2020.07.006
0889-857X/20/© 2020 Elsevier Inc. All rights reserved.
rheumatic.theclinics.com

Table 1
Summary of rheumatic disease epidemiology

Condition	Prevalence Summary	Prevalence Details	Incidence Summary	Incidence Details	Phenotype Summary
Rheumatoid arthritis	High	1.4%–7.1%[1,9,10]	High	2–10 times US white[1] Higher in relatives of people with RA[3]	High prevalence of seropositivity for RF, CCP, ANA[1,11,12] More nodules and erosions[1] Earlier age of onset[11] More large joint involvement[11]
Spondyloarthritis	High	2.5% overall[2] 1.5–2.7 times higher in First Nations vs non-First Nations in Alberta[10]	Unknown	—	High prevalence of HLA B27[14] Undifferentiated and reactive arthritis more common than AS[2] More severe disease in men[19]
Juvenile idiopathic arthritis	Probably high	79 per 100,000[23]	Unknown	—	Enthesitis-related arthritis overrepresented[23]
Systemic lupus erythematosus	High	270.6 per 100,000 women and 53.8 per 100,000 men[28]	High	7.4 per 100,000 person-years overall[28]	Early age of onset[25,33] Arthritis common[13,17,25,28] Renal disease may be more common[28]
Mixed connective tissue disease	Probably high	6.4 per 100,000[35]	Unknown	—	Synovitis and Raynaud most common manifestations[35]
Systemic sclerosis	Probably high	66 per 100,000 in 1 Oklahoma tribe[36] 47 per 100,000 in First Nations in Alberta[26]	Unknown	—	—
Sjogren syndrome	Maybe high	High proportion of cases in a cohort were AI but prevalence unknown[37]	Unknown	—	—
Inflammatory myopathy	Unknown	25 per 100,000 in First Nations in Alberta (low)[38] Concern of possible higher rates of statin-associated autoimmune myopathy in US AI/AN populations[39]	Unknown	—	—

Osteoarthritis	High	16.1 per 100 (2× as common as non-First Nations in Alberta)[43]	Unknown	—	Higher all-cause hospitalization rates, but lower rates of specialty care and joint replacement[43]
Crystal-associated arthritis	Low	0.8 per 100 First Nations (vs 1.2 per 100 non-First Nations) in Alberta[10]	Unknown	—
Self-reported arthritis	High	24.4% in AI/AN in NHIS in United States, vs 22.6% in non-Hispanic whites[44]	Unknown	—

This article provides an overview of the epidemiology of rheumatic diseases in INA populations. A systematic review was recently published on this topic,[5] and this article includes key studies available before that systematic review, as well as more recently published literature. When discussing future research directions, the importance of community engagement and a summary of past community engagement in rheumatic disease research are also highlighted. Systematic reviews have also been published recently describing rheumatic disease phenotype and outcomes,[6] health care utilization,[7] and mortality[8] in indigenous populations.

EPIDEMIOLOGY OF RHEUMATIC DISEASES
Rheumatoid Arthritis

A high prevalence of RA has been described in multiple INA populations, ranging from 1.4% to 7.1% in a 2005 review, compared with less than 1% in the general population.[1] The incidence of RA has not been studied as frequently, but ranged from more than 2 times expected to up to 10 times expected in 2 studies.[1] The prevalence of RA in different INA populations has varied, some of which can be attributed to differences in population prevalence and some to differences in study design. Since the review of this topic in 2005, two additional studies confirmed a high prevalence of RA. In Manitoba, Canada, RA was twice as common in First Nations compared with non-First Nations people based on claims data.[9] In Alberta, Canada, the prevalence of RA in First Nations people was 3.2%, three times higher than in non-First Nations people.[10] A recent study of a cohort of relatives of INA people with RA, who are at higher risk than the general population, found the incidence of inflammatory arthritis to be 9.2 per 1000 person-years.[3]

Several studies have described the phenotype of RA in INA populations. Older studies documented a high prevalence of seropositivity for rheumatoid factor (RF) (>90%) and antinuclear antibody (ANA) (>50%), with increased likelihood of rheumatoid nodules and erosions.[1] More recent studies have confirmed the high proportion of cases with positive RF and ANA[11] and described more than 80% seropositivity for anticyclic citrullinated peptide (CCP).[12] An exception was a study of Oklahoma tribal populations that found anti-CCP positivity in only 55% of patients with RA and RF positivity in only 58%, although ANA positivity was still common (62.5%).[13] An earlier age of onset and high frequency of large joint involvement have been described.[11]

Spondyloarthritis

Studies of spondyloarthropathy in the AN population in the 1980s found high rates of HLA B27 positivity in the population (25%–40%), but lower than expected prevalence of ankylosing spondylitis (AS).[14–17] Because a large proportion of cases was consistent with undifferentiated spondyloarthropathy rather than AS, studies were repeated in the 1990s with a broader set of criteria. In AN people in 2 regions of Northern and Western Alaska, the overall prevalence of spondyloarthropathy was 2.5%,[2] in comparison to approximately 0.9% to 1.4% in the US population,[18] including a high prevalence of reactive arthritis (1.0%) and undifferentiated spondyloarthropathy (1.3%), with AS being less common (0.4%).[2] Psoriatic arthritis was rare, with a prevalence of less than 0.1%.[2] A subsequent study identified more severe disease in AN men than women.[19] Older studies in Canadian Inuit and Indian populations also identified high prevalence of spondyloarthropathy.[20,21] A more recent study in Alberta, Canada using claims-based data found the prevalence of psoriatic disease (psoriasis and psoriatic arthritis) to be 0.3% in the First Nations population, with a standardized rate ratio (SRR) of 1.5 when compared with the non-First Nations population.[10] This same study found AS prevalence to be 0.6%, with SRR of 2.7 in the First Nations compared with non-First Nations population.[10]

Juvenile Idiopathic Arthritis

Two studies using the older juvenile rheumatoid arthritis (JRA) classification criteria found a high prevalence of JRA in 2 Indian Health Service (IHS) regions[22] and in Southeast Alaska.[17] A recent study in Alaska using the International League Against Rheumatism classification criteria found the prevalence of JIA in AN children to be 79 per 100,000, higher than the reported prevalence of 50 per 100,000 in a recent study in Olmsted County, Minnesota.[23] In this study, although oligoarthritis was the most common form of JIA, enthesitis-related arthritis made up a higher proportion of cases (24%) than expected (1%–3%), and HLA B27 was positive in more than half of the children who were tested.[23]

Systemic Lupus Erythematosus

The incidence and prevalence of SLE were higher than expected in many studies of INA populations using regional or administrative data before 2013.[17,24–26] A national study published in 2013 using data from the US Medicaid population confirmed that incidence and prevalence of SLE were high in individuals identified as Native American, but not as high as in the US black population.[27] The CDC funded 5 population-based lupus registries, designed to address the limitations of epidemiologic data for SLE in multiple populations in the United States. The 5 registries used similar population-based surveillance methods, with medical record abstraction for verification of each case. The IHS registry catchment area included 3 administrative areas, Alaska, Phoenix, and Oklahoma City. Data from the 5 registries have been published, with the highest prevalence of SLE found in AI/AN populations in the IHS lupus registry.[28–32] Incidence of SLE was also high in AI/AN populations, but with wider confidence intervals. A metaanalysis has been conducted to estimate the prevalence of SLE in the United States and the number of people living with SLE in the United States, combining data from the 4 state-based registries and comparing it to the AI/AN prevalence determined by the IHS registry.[4] The highest prevalence of SLE was in AI/AN women (270.6 per 100,000) and men (53.8), compared with the next highest rates in black women (230.9) and black men (26.7).[4]

In INA populations, a few studies have described a younger mean age of onset of SLE.[25,33] Several studies have described arthritis as a more common manifestation of SLE than in other populations (>80%).[13,17,25,28] Renal disease, a predictor of higher mortality, has been reported in about 40% of INA people with SLE in several studies, a prevalence that is similar to that reported in blacks with SLE and higher than what has been reported in whites.[28]

Other Systemic Rheumatic Disease

A study in the 1980s suggested a high rate of overlap syndromes in INA populations in Canada.[34] A recent report using data collected in the IHS lupus registry found the age-adjusted prevalence of mixed connective tissue disease in AI/AN populations in the United States to be 6.4 per 100,000 by the primary definition, which was higher than the prevalence in a comparable study in Norway (3.8),[35] with no data available for comparison in North America. A study in the 1990s identified a very high prevalence of systemic sclerosis in 1 tribe in southeastern Oklahoma (66 per 100,000 overall).[36] Since then, 1 study found higher rates of systemic sclerosis in First Nations compared with non-First Nations people in Alberta, Canada, especially in women over the age of 45.[26] A recent study found an overrepresentation of AI patients in a

Sjogren syndrome cohort, leading the investigators to suspect a higher prevalence of Sjogren syndrome in this population.[37] Autoimmune inflammatory myopathy prevalence was studied in Alberta, Canada, with similar prevalence found in the First Nations compared with non-First Nations population.[38] Of note, the IHS issued a drug safety alert in January 2019 noting a high number of cases of statin-associated autoimmune myopathy, with plans for an epidemiologic investigation by the Food and Drug Administration.[39] Finally, a few studies of vasculitis are available. These studies have documented high rates of hepatitis B–associated polyarteritis nodosa in AN people in a region with high rates of hepatitis B infection,[40] low hospitalization rates for Kawasaki syndrome in children in IHS facilities,[41] and low incidence of biopsy-proven giant cell arteritis in AN people.[42]

Osteoarthritis and Self-Reported Arthritis

A recent study in Alberta, Canada found that osteoarthritis was twice as common in First Nations compared with non-First Nations people based on administrative claims data.[43] Self-reported arthritis is a common measure of the burden of arthritis in populations in national or state-based surveys. In the United States from 2013 to 2015, the age-adjusted prevalence of self-reported doctor-diagnosed arthritis in the National Health Interview Survey (NHIS) was 24.4% in AI/AN people, compared with 22.6% in non-Hispanic whites, with lower rates in other racial/ethnic groups.[44] A population-based cohort of AI/AN people in Alaska and the Southwestern United States found a higher age-adjusted prevalence of self-reported arthritis in AN people (26.1%) than in the general US population by NHIS at the time (21.5%) or in AI people in the Southwestern United States (16.5%).[45]

Crystal-Induced Arthritis

A few studies suggest a low prevalence of crystal-induced arthritis in INA populations, in contrast to indigenous populations of New Zealand, where a high prevalence of gout has been described.[46] A study in the 1980s found a low prevalence of gout (0.3%) in a Northwestern AN population.[15] A recent study using administrative claims data found lower prevalence of crystal-induced arthritis in First Nations compared with non-First Nations populations in Alberta, Canada, with an SRR of 0.7.[10]

RISK FACTORS FOR RHEUMATIC DISEASE

The risk of rheumatic disease is based on a combination of many genetic and environmental factors. Genetic factors have been studied more often and are summarized in later discussion. Environmental factors, such as tobacco use, stress and adverse childhood experiences, infections, the microbiome, socioeconomic status, and epigenetic factors, are all likely key risk factors, but few have been studied. In a study of the incidence of inflammatory arthritis in family members of INA people with RA, history of smoking was common (>75%) in both progressors and nonprogressors, with no statistically significant difference between groups.[3]

Genetic Risk Factors for Rheumatoid Arthritis and Spondyloarthritis

A unique shared epitope allele (HLA DRB1*1402) was identified with a high frequency in INA populations.[1] A metaanalysis of data from 3 INA populations in the United States confirmed an association of HLA DRB1*1402 and RA.[47] A recent study provided confirmation of the association of this allele with RA in INA populations and additional information on the mechanism of risk, related to the capacity to present citrullinated peptide antigens and T-cell expansion.[48]

As a possible explanation for high rates of spondyloarthritis, the prevalence of HLA B27 was found to be elevated in many INA populations, ranging from 25% to 40%,[14] in contrast to approximately 6% in the US population.[49]

FUTURE DIRECTIONS AND THE IMPORTANCE OF COMMUNITY ENGAGEMENT IN RHEUMATIC DISEASE RESEARCH WITH INDIGENOUS NORTH AMERICAN POPULATIONS

As described above, there are few studies of risk factors for rheumatic disease specifically in INA populations. Although more research is needed, it is important that researchers interested in studying rheumatic diseases in indigenous populations understand the community context and unique ethical considerations. Misconduct and misuse of research data and specimens have occurred too frequently, often in the context of secondary use without knowledge or consent of participants. The most recent widely known episode occurred when members of the Havasupai tribe were recruited for a study of diabetes, but with secondary use of specimens for genetic research on topics that were not acceptable to tribal members.[50] In order to avoid researcher misinterpretation of research findings or stigmatization of populations with high rates of disease, engagement of indigenous communities in research is critical. A systematic review was recently published evaluating the degree of community engagement in arthritis research.[51] Community engagement was most common during the data collection stage of arthritis research, with few studies engaging communities during the inception or interpretation and dissemination stage of research. Most community engagement was at the lower end of the spectrum, with few studies including meaningful community engagement. Processes that promote meaningful community engagement are recommended for arthritis studies in indigenous populations.[51]

SUMMARY

The prevalence of many rheumatic diseases is high in INA populations, especially RA, SLE, and spondyloarthritis, which have been studied most extensively. The risk factors underlying the high burden of rheumatic diseases in INA populations are not fully known. Understanding the epidemiology of rheumatic disease in INA populations is important for clinicians, health systems, and communities. Providing education to these stakeholders about the burden of disease and improving access to specialist care in these populations may help identify rheumatic diseases earlier and improve outcomes. Finally, community engagement in rheumatic disease research in INA populations is critical to ensure that research is culturally relevant and has the potential to benefit INA communities.

DISCLOSURE

The authors have nothing to disclose.

REFERENCES

1. Ferucci ED, Templin DW, Lanier AP. Rheumatoid arthritis in American Indians and Alaska Natives: a review of the literature. Semin Arthritis Rheum 2005;34(4): 662–7.

2. Boyer GS, Templin DW, Cornoni-Huntley JC, et al. Prevalence of spondyloarthropathies in Alaskan Eskimos. J Rheumatol 1994;21(12):2292–7.

3. Tanner S, Dufault B, Smolik I, et al. A prospective study of the development of inflammatory arthritis in the family members of indigenous North American people with rheumatoid arthritis. Arthritis Rheumatol 2019;71(9):1494–503.

4. Somers E, Wang L, McCune WJ, et al. Prevalence of Systemic Lupus Erythematosus in the United States: Preliminary Estimates from a Meta-Analysis of the Centers for Disease Control and Prevention Lupus Registries [abstract]. Arthritis Rheumatol 2019;71(Suppl 10). Available at: https://acrabstracts.org/abstract/prevalence-of-systemic-lupus-erythematosus-in-the-united-states-preliminary-estimates-from-a-meta-analysis-of-the-centers-for-disease-control-and-prevention-lupus-registries/. Accessed July 27, 2020.

5. McDougall C, Hurd K, Barnabe C. Systematic review of rheumatic disease epidemiology in the indigenous populations of Canada, the United States, Australia, and New Zealand. Semin Arthritis Rheum 2017;46(5):675–86.

6. Hurd K, Barnabe C. Systematic review of rheumatic disease phenotypes and outcomes in the Indigenous populations of Canada, the USA, Australia and New Zealand. Rheumatol Int 2017;37(4):503–21.

7. Loyola-Sanchez A, Hurd K, Barnabe C. Healthcare utilization for arthritis by indigenous populations of Australia, Canada, New Zealand, and the United States: a systematic review. Semin Arthritis Rheum 2017;46(5):665–74.

8. Hurd K, Barnabe C. Mortality causes and outcomes in indigenous populations of Canada, the United States, and Australia with rheumatic disease: a systematic review. Semin Arthritis Rheum 2018;47(4):586–92.

9. Barnabe C, Elias B, Bartlett J, et al. Arthritis in aboriginal manitobans: evidence for a high burden of disease. J Rheumatol 2008;35(6):1145–50.

10. Barnabe C, Jones CA, Bernatsky S, et al. Inflammatory arthritis prevalence and health services use in the First Nations and non-First Nations populations of Alberta, Canada. Arthritis Care Res (Hoboken) 2017;69(4):467–74.

11. Peschken CA, Hitchon CA, Robinson DB, et al. Rheumatoid arthritis in a North American Native population: longitudinal followup and comparison with a white population. J Rheumatol 2010;37(8):1589–95.

12. El-Gabalawy HS, Robinson DB, Hart D, et al. Immunogenetic risks of anti-cyclical citrullinated peptide antibodies in a North American Native population with rheumatoid arthritis and their first-degree relatives. J Rheumatol 2009;36(6):1130–5.

13. Gaddy JR, Vista ES, Robertson JM, et al. Rheumatic disease among Oklahoma tribal populations: a cross-sectional study. J Rheumatol 2012;39(10):1934–41.

14. Hansen JA, Lanier AP, Nisperos B, et al. The HLA system in Inupiat and Central Yupik Alaskan Eskimos. Hum Immunol 1986;16(4):315–28.

15. Boyer GS, Lanier AP, Templin DW. Prevalence rates of spondyloarthropathies, rheumatoid arthritis, and other rheumatic disorders in an Alaskan Inupiat Eskimo population. J Rheumatol 1988;15(4):678–83.

16. Boyer GS, Lanier AP, Templin DW, et al. Spondyloarthropathy and rheumatoid arthritis in Alaskan Yupik Eskimos. J Rheumatol 1990;17(4):489–96.

17. Boyer GS, Templin DW, Lanier AP. Rheumatic diseases in Alaskan Indians of the southeast coast: high prevalence of rheumatoid arthritis and systemic lupus erythematosus. J Rheumatol 1991;18(10):1477–84.

18. Reveille JD, Witter JP, Weisman MH. Prevalence of axial spondylarthritis in the United States: estimates from a cross-sectional survey. Arthritis Care Res (Hoboken) 2012;64(6):905–10.

19. Boyer GS, Templin DW, Bowler A, et al. Spondyloarthropathy in the community: differences in severity and disease expression in Alaskan Eskimo men and women. J Rheumatol 2000;27(1):170–6.

20. Oen K, Postl B, Chalmers IM, et al. Rheumatic diseases in an Inuit population. Arthritis Rheum 1986;29(1):65–74.
21. Robinson HS, Gofton JP, Price GE. A study of rheumatic disease in a Canadian Indian population. Ann Rheum Dis 1963;22:232–6.
22. Mauldin J, Cameron HD, Jeanotte D, et al. Chronic arthritis in children and adolescents in two Indian health service user populations. BMC Musculoskelet Disord 2004;5:30.
23. Khodra B, Stevens A, Ferucci ED. Prevalence of Juvenile Idiopathic Arthritis in the Alaska Native Population. Arthritis Care Res (Hoboken) 2019 May 31. https://doi.org/10.1002/acr.23997. Online ahead of print.
24. Acers TE, Acers-Warn A. Incidence patterns of immunogenetic diseases in the North American Indians. J Okla State Med Assoc 1994;87(7):309–14.
25. Peschken CA, Esdaile JM. Systemic lupus erythematosus in North American Indians: a population based study. J Rheumatol 2000;27(8):1884–91.
26. Barnabe C, Joseph L, Belisle P, et al. Prevalence of systemic lupus erythematosus and systemic sclerosis in the First Nations population of Alberta, Canada. Arthritis Care Res (Hoboken) 2012;64(1):138–43.
27. Feldman CH, Hiraki LT, Liu J, et al. Epidemiology and sociodemographics of systemic lupus erythematosus and lupus nephritis among US adults with Medicaid coverage, 2000-2004. Arthritis Rheum 2013;65(3):753–63.
28. Ferucci ED, Johnston JM, Gaddy JR, et al. Prevalence and incidence of systemic lupus erythematosus in a population-based registry of American Indian and Alaska Native people, 2007-2009. Arthritis Rheumatol 2014;66(9):2494–502.
29. Lim SS, Bayakly AR, Helmick CG, et al. The incidence and prevalence of systemic lupus erythematosus, 2002-2004: the Georgia Lupus Registry. Arthritis Rheum 2013;66(2):357–68.
30. Somers EC, Marder W, Cagnoli P, et al. Population-based incidence and prevalence of systemic lupus erythematosus: the Michigan Lupus Epidemiology & Surveillance (MILES) Program. Arthritis Rheumatol 2014 Feb;66(2):369–78. https://doi.org/10.1002/art.38238.
31. Izmirly PM, Wan I, Sahl S, et al. The incidence and prevalence of systemic lupus erythematosus in New York County (Manhattan), New York: the Manhattan Lupus Surveillance Program. Arthritis Rheumatol 2017;69(10):2006–17.
32. Dall'Era M, Cisternas MG, Snipes K, et al. The incidence and prevalence of systemic lupus erythematosus in San Francisco County, California: the California Lupus Surveillance Project. Arthritis Rheumatol 2017;69(10):1996–2005.
33. Kheir JM, Guthridge CJ, Johnston JR, et al. Unique clinical characteristics, autoantibodies and medication use in Native American patients with systemic lupus erythematosus. Lupus Sci Med 2018;5(1):e000247.
34. Atkins C, Reuffel L, Roddy J, et al. Rheumatic disease in the Nuu-Chah-Nulth native Indians of the Pacific Northwest. J Rheumatol 1988;15(4):684–90.
35. Ferucci ED, Johnston JM, Gordon C, et al. Prevalence of mixed connective tissue disease in a population-based registry of American Indian/Alaska Native people in 2007. Arthritis Care Res (Hoboken) 2016;69(8):1271–5.
36. Arnett FC, Howard RF, Tan F, et al. Increased prevalence of systemic sclerosis in a Native American tribe in Oklahoma. Association with an Amerindian HLA haplotype. Arthritis Rheum 1996;39(8):1362–70.
37. Scofield RH, Sharma R, Pezant N, et al. American Indians have a higher risk of Sjogren's syndrome and more disease activity than caucasians and African-Americans. Arthritis Care Res (Hoboken) 2019 Jun;14. https://doi.org/10.1002/acr.24003. Online ahead of print.

38. Barnabe C, Joseph L, Belisle P, et al. Prevalence of autoimmune inflammatory myopathy in the First Nations population of Alberta, Canada. Arthritis Care Res (Hoboken) 2012;64(11):1715–9.

39. Service IH. Drug safety alert: statin-associated autoimmune myopathy 2019. Available at: https://www.ihs.gov/sites/nptc/themes/responsive2017/display_objects/documents/guidance/NPTC-Drug-Safety-Alert-Statin-Associated-Autoimmune-Myopathy.pdf. Accessed February 28, 2020.

40. McMahon BJ, Bender TR, Templin DW, et al. Vasculitis in Eskimos living in an area hyperendemic for hepatitis B. JAMA 1980;244(19):2180–2.

41. Holman RC, Belay ED, Clarke MJ, et al. Kawasaki syndrome among American Indian and Alaska Native children, 1980 through 1995. Pediatr Infect Dis J 1999; 18(5):451–5.

42. Mader TH, Werner RP, Chamberlain DG, et al. Giant cell arteritis in Alaska Natives. Can J Ophthalmol 2009;44(1):53–6.

43. Barnabe C, Hemmelgarn B, Jones CA, et al. Imbalance of prevalence and specialty care for osteoarthritis for First Nations people in Alberta, Canada. J Rheumatol 2015;42(2):323–8.

44. Barbour KE, Helmick CG, Boring M, et al. Vital signs: prevalence of doctor-diagnosed arthritis and arthritis-attributable activity limitation - United States, 2013-2015. MMWR Morb Mortal Wkly Rep 2017;66(9):246–53.

45. Ferucci ED, Schumacher MC, Lanier AP, et al. Arthritis prevalence and associations in American Indian and Alaska Native people. Arthritis Care Res 2008;59(8):1128–36.

46. Stamp LK, Wells JE, Pitama S, et al. Hyperuricaemia and gout in New Zealand rural and urban Maori and non-Maori communities. Intern Med J 2013;43(6):678–84.

47. Williams RC, Jacobsson LT, Knowler WC, et al. Meta-analysis reveals association between most common class II haplotype in full-heritage Native Americans and rheumatoid arthritis. Hum Immunol 1995;42(1):90–4.

48. Scally SW, Law SC, Ting YT, et al. Molecular basis for increased susceptibility of Indigenous North Americans to seropositive rheumatoid arthritis. Ann Rheum Dis 2017;76(11):1915–23.

49. Reveille JD, Hirsch R, Dillon CF, et al. The prevalence of HLA-B27 in the US: data from the US National Health and Nutrition Examination Survey, 2009. Arthritis Rheum 2012;64(5):1407–11.

50. Mello MM, Wolf LE. The Havasupai Indian tribe case–lessons for research involving stored biologic samples. N Engl J Med 2010;363(3):204–7.

51. Lin CY, Loyola-Sanchez A, Hurd K, et al. Characterization of indigenous community engagement in arthritis studies conducted in Canada, United States of America, Australia and New Zealand. Semin Arthritis Rheum 2019;49(1):145–55.

Disparities in Childhood-Onset Lupus

Tamar B. Rubinstein, MD, MS[a],*, Andrea M. Knight, MD, MSCE[b]

KEYWORDS

- Pediatric • Lupus • Disparities • Race • Ethnicity • Socioeconomic • Geographic
- Access

KEY POINTS

- There are known disparities in the prevalence of childhood-onset systemic lupus erythematosus (SLE), disease severity, physical and mental morbidity, and mortality across racial/ethnic groups.
- Although health care quality for pediatric patients with SLE varies by socioeconomic status and accessibility of pediatric rheumatologists, there are significant gaps in the literature regarding the impact of socioeconomic status on health outcomes.
- Further studies are needed to better understand specific drivers for disparate outcomes for patients with childhood-onset SLE, and to develop effective interventions for eliminating health inequity.

INTRODUCTION

Systemic lupus erythematosus (SLE) occurring in childhood, as in adults, is a chronic, autoimmune disease that has the potential to involve any organ system. In children and youth with childhood-onset SLE (cSLE), however, the most severe forms of SLE, namely life-threatening renal or central nervous system (CNS) disease, occur more frequently.[1] Individuals with cSLE are at risk of stroke, end-stage renal disease (ESRD), and early death.[2–4]

Similar to adult-onset disease, cSLE does not affect populations equally. Higher prevalence rates have been reported in several racial and ethnic minorities, most notably in Native American and First Nation Canadians, black, Latino, and Asian people.[5–8]

Furthermore, disparities have been observed in outcomes of cSLE, care delivery, and SLE-related comorbidities, including mental health disorders. These disparities may be along the lines of race/ethnicity, income, and geography. Despite this, the

[a] Department of Pediatrics, Division of Pediatric Rheumatology, Children's Hospital at Montefiore/Albert Einstein College of Medicine, 3415 Bainbridge Avenue, Bronx, NY 10467, USA;
[b] Division of Rheumatology, The Hospital for Sick Children, 555 University Avenue, Toronto, Ontario M5G 1X8, Canada
* Corresponding author.
E-mail address: trubinst@montefiore.org
Twitter: @tamarpedsrheum (T.B.R.)

Rheum Dis Clin N Am 46 (2020) 661–672
https://doi.org/10.1016/j.rdc.2020.07.007
0889-857X/20/© 2020 Elsevier Inc. All rights reserved.

understanding of disparities affecting patients with cSLE is limited by a dearth of large studies with diverse demographics and a paucity of studies that examined differences across demographics.

In this review, the authors present the current knowledge regarding disparities in cSLE and related outcomes and the gaps in knowledge that require further investigation. In this review of the literature on disparities in cSLE, the authors used a broad definition of health disparities, consistent with Health People 2020, as "a particular type of health difference that is closely linked with social, economic, and/or environmental disadvantage."[9]

DISPARITIES IN PREVALENCE OF CHILDHOOD-ONSET SYSTEMIC LUPUS ERYTHEMATOSUS

Populations across the globe are not at equal risk of developing SLE. Studies that have been conducted looking at prevalence discrepancies across populations in cSLE show similar trends to what has been described in adult-onset SLE. Native American/American Indian children have the highest documented prevalence rates globally of cSLE. Among child Medicaid beneficiaries in the United States, Native American children are more than 3 times as likely to develop cSLE that other US race/ethnicities with prevalence rates of 13.4 per 100,000.[5] These prevalence rates have been corroborated in studies of prevalence rates among Native American children seen by Indian Health Services.[6] Children of First-Nation populations in Canada also appear to be at greater risk of developing cSLE than other Canadians. British Columbia First Nations children have a prevalence rate of 8.8 per 100,000 for SLE compared with 3.3 per 100,000 in the general population.[10]

Asian populations, both in Asia and across the globe, also exhibit higher prevalence rates of cSLE than the prevalence rates documented in European populations[11,12] and in general US[13] and Canadian populations.[14] Chinese children from Taiwan have a prevalence of 6.3 per 100,000.[7]

Although SLE prevalence rates in New Zealand and Australia are much lower than the United States and Canada, children of indigenous populations of New Zealand (Maori) are twice as likely to have SLE as their counterparts of European descent in New Zealand.[15] Rates of SLE in Aboriginal and Torres Strait Islander children of Australia are 4 times that of the general pediatric population of Australia.[16]

In the United States and Canada, single-center studies from large urban cities indicate that Asian, black, and Latino/Hispanic children have higher prevalence rates of SLE than white children,[14] similar to adult-onset SLE. In particular, black SLE patients are among the youngest diagnosed with SLE and disproportionately represent cSLE populations, even in comparison to what is expected from the increased rates of cSLE overall.[8]

Finally, for large populations in developing countries, the epidemiology of cSLE is largely unknown. In many lower- and middle-income countries in Africa and Asia, with large populations and very few pediatric rheumatologists, delays in diagnosis and delays in access to care have been described. Likely a large proportion of cases in these underserved countries are being missed. In South Africa, for instance, the large burden of infectious disease, including human immunodeficiency virus, and trauma is noted to overwhelm underresourced medical systems, challenging care for chronic pediatric disease.[17] Similar challenges have been described in India, with regard to the care of children with SLE.[18]

DISPARITIES IN DISEASE MANIFESTATIONS AND SEVERITY

Several early studies that examined differences in SLE disease manifestations and reported data on demographic groups of cSLE patients had either too few minority patients[19] or too few numbers overall to fully investigate differences across demographics. However, even among these, it is evident that some of the most severe SLE manifestations, such as lupus nephritis (LN) and CNS lupus, are more prevalent among black and Hispanic patients.[14,19]

Recent studies, including two from large academic centers in Canada[14] and the United Kingdom,[20] show more definitively increased rates of LN in nonwhite SLE children. Although the UK study only reported race/ethnicity dichotomously as white/nonwhite,[20] others reported race-specific rates of LN in black children with SLE between 36% and 64%[14,21,22] and 66% in Asian children.[14] The largest cohort to date representing black children in the United States is from the first iteration of the SLE registry of the Childhood Arthritis and Rheumatology Research Alliance (CARRA Legacy Registry), which includes approximately 1000 patients from 60 CARRA sites across the United States, 35% of whom are black.[21] The rate of biopsy-confirmed LN in black CARRA Registry patients is 42%,[21] similar to the overall rate of biopsy-proven LN in the total CARRA Legacy Registry (43%).[23] Lewandowski and colleagues[21] compared the CARRA Registry patients with a cohort of mainly nonwhite patients of African descent (92%) from South Africa and found that patients represented in the South African cohort had notably higher rates of biopsy-proven LN (61%). This cohort, the PULSE cohort, is a retrospective cohort of pediatric SLE patients developed from records at 3 hospital centers in Cape Town, South Africa who presented from 1988 to 2012.

A study from China found LN in 61% of children with cSLE.[7] In contrast, in a cohort from Singapore, which was largely of Chinese ethnicity, the rate of LN was 41%.[24] In a cohort of 33 children from Trinidad, the rate of renal disease (not biopsy proven) was 64%.[25] The highest rates of LN documented were in small cohorts of cSLE patients from Egypt (88%) and Turkey (86%), but these rates are likely biased based on the composition of these cohorts of patients referred to pediatric nephrology (despite potential absence of resources in pediatric rheumatology).[26,27]

Less is known about neuropsychiatric manifestations across demographics in cSLE. Rates of CNS disease in cSLE vary greatly between studies, and few studies reported rates across race/ethnicity. Rates reported range between 24% and 27% from cohorts from Canada, United States, and China, and up to 95% from 1 cohort from New Mexico with most being Hispanic patients.[28] These rates are likely due as much to the differences in definition and attribution (specifically for symptoms of lupus headache, cognitive dysfunction, and mood disorder) as they are to variance among prevalence rates in differing populations. Hiraki and colleagues[14] found that black children with cSLE had the highest proportion of CNS disease with 32% affected, compared with 24% in white patients and significantly higher than the 18% Asian children with SLE.

In the largest cohort to date to study cardiac manifestations of cSLE, from the United States, Chang and colleagues[29] found that black race was associated with an incident rate ratio of 6.6 compared with white race. Although cardiac manifestations were reported with a similar frequency in the PULSE cohort from South Africa, they had worse severity than the US cohort described by Chang and colleagues.[30]

DISPARITIES IN MORBIDITY AND MORTALITY

Among sources of organ damage from SLE in childhood and young adults, renal damage and specifically ESRD are best studied. In a large US study that looked across ages, black SLE patients were at the highest risk for ESRD among young people with LN.[31] From 1995 to 2006, rates of ESRD among black LN patients have increased, as have rates of ESRD among LN patients ages 5 to 39.[32] Among pediatric LN patients with ESRD captured by the US Renal Data System, black children were half as likely to receive transplants as white children and almost twice as likely to die. Hispanic patients were also less likely to receive transplants than non-Hispanic patients. Regional disparities were also found, because children in the southern United States were less likely to receive transplants than children in the northwest and western United States.[31] Outside of the United States, high rates of ESRD from LN were described in the South African PULSE cohort (13%).[21]

Osteoporosis/osteopenia is another form of SLE-related damage. In a preliminarily study, disparities in osteoporosis/osteopenia by race/ethnicity were not evident.[33]

SLE-related damage, in general, measured by Systemic Lupus International Collaborating Clinics SLE Damage Index (SLICC SDI) also showed no race/ethnicity disparities in a study from British Columbia, largely of white and Asian patients, and with no black or Hispanic patients[34] and from a multinational study of cSLE, including centers from North America, Europe, and Asia.[35] In contrast, a significantly higher percentage of children from the South African PULSE cohort had evidence of damage on SLICC SDI compared with those from a US cohort (from the CARRA Legacy Registry), 63% versus 23%.[21] Within the CARRA Legacy Registry, poverty, and not race/ethnicity, was associated with worse disability.[36]

Although decreases in mortality in cSLE have been described over the past 20 years, mortality still remains significant, specifically because of ESRD. cSLE patients with ESRD have twice the risk of death compared with other pediatric ESRD patients.[2]

A recent large national study of US pediatric patients with SLE showed regional and racial disparities in mortality. Black children and children from the southern US region had twice the risk of death with inpatient hospitalizations, compared with white children and children from the northeastern US.[4]

In another study that was not designed or powered to find significant differences in mortality, the proportion of deaths seen in minority race/ethnicities, and most notably in black children with SLE, was outsized.[14] In a small Trinidadian cohort of cSLE, East Indian and mixed race children had the highest mortalities (higher than black children or children of African descent).[25]

DISPARITIES IN MENTAL HEALTH AND HEALTH-RELATED QUALITY OF LIFE

Although a cross-sectional study of depression and anxiety in US youth with cSLE found that youth of nonwhite race were more likely to have symptoms of depression,[37] a large study of Medicaid-enrolled cSLE youth found that black children with cSLE were significantly less likely to be diagnosed with anxiety or depression, and less likely to be treated with anxiolytics.[22]

Specific disparities around mental health diagnosis and treatment among lower-income US black children with cSLE may have long-lasting effects on not only the mental health but also on the physical health of this population, given observed associations between mental health symptoms and aspects of self-care, such as medication adherence.[38]

Studies of associations between health-related quality of life (HRQOL) and race/ethnicity in cSLE populations have been inconsistent. In studies including US populations, black race[39] and nonwhite race[40] were risk factors for lower HRQOL measures, although a Canadian study found the opposite, with children identifying as white more likely to report worse HRQOL.[41]

DISPARITIES IN HEALTH CARE QUALITY AND UTILIZATION

Disparities between younger and older adult SLE patients have been identified with regards to quality of care. Young adult patients aged 18 to 34 are less likely than older adults to receive care that meets quality metrics related to SLE care, including pneumococcal vaccination, medication toxicity monitoring, and cardiovascular monitoring.[42] However, few studies have examined quality metrics across demographics, specifically among cSLE patients.

Among Medicaid-enrolled US youth with SLE, black, Hispanic, and "other" nonwhite races have higher rates of glucocorticoid use,[22] although this may be a result of differences in disease severity or activity. Similarly, greater cost for inpatient hospitalization is associated with male gender and black race among US children hospitalized with SLE.[43]

Disparities During Transition to Adulthood

The transition period between pediatric and adult health care models is a time of particular vulnerability to poor outcomes and barriers to quality care and access to care. Thus, in cSLE, this is a period of special concern. Limited studies have investigated potential race/ethnicity disparities during transition. A recent study of a large administrative database of youth on private insurance found that there were no differences among SLE youth in the rates of successful transfer to adult rheumatology by race/ethnicity. Neither were there differences in health care utilization.[44] A smaller study of patients from Boston found that white race and low education were associated with missed appointments during transition.[45] In adolescents and young adults with chronic diseases, living in higher-income neighborhoods is associated with transition readiness.[46]

Causes and contributors to these disparities in cSLE in US populations have yet to be investigated. A qualitative study in South Africa of adult caregivers and medical providers caring for children with SLE explored barriers to seeking and receiving care for cSLE, and how they may contribute to poor outcomes observed in this population of SLE patients. Major barriers included severe financial difficulties for families (18% of families came from households without running water or electricity), social stigma related to a chronic diagnosis, lack of trained staff in pediatric rheumatology, and prior misdiagnosis.[17]

Access to pediatric rheumatologists may drive some disparities in US populations as well. A study of SLE patients enrolled in the CARRA Legacy Registry found that location in a state with a high density of pediatric rheumatologists was a predictor for being seen expeditiously (within the first month from symptom onset), whereas being from a low-income household was a predictor for severe delay (seen ≥1 year from symptom onset).[47]

POTENTIAL CONTRIBUTORS TO DISPARITIES

Several potential contributors to disparities in cSLE have yet to be fully investigated. In **Fig. 1**, the authors describe different factors related to social disadvantage, health care systems and access, family environment and resources, and individual patient treatment that may lead to inequities in care for youth with cSLE. This conceptual framework is based on social-ecological models of health, such as Bronfenbrenner's, used in other disciplines to study health disparities.[48]

Although challenges of caring for patients with cSLE by a small pediatric rheumatology workforce have been well described, regarding areas of the globe and states within the United States that lack access to specialists, the impact of the limitations

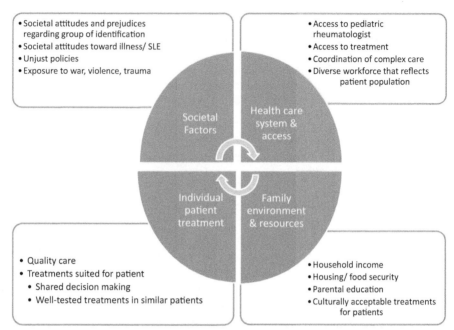

- Societal attitudes and prejudices regarding group of identification
- Societal attitudes toward illness/ SLE
- Unjust policies
- Exposure to war, violence, trauma

- Access to pediatric rheumatologist
- Access to treatment
- Coordination of complex care
- Diverse workforce that reflects patient population

Societal Factors

Health care system & access

Individual patient treatment

Family environment & resources

- Quality care
- Treatments suited for patient
- Shared decision making
- Well-tested treatments in similar patients

- Household income
- Housing/ food security
- Parental education
- Culturally acceptable treatments for patients

Fig. 1. Modified social-ecological model of contributors to health disparities and health equity in cSLE. Potential contributors to health disparities in cSLE related to societal, health system and health access, family, and individual patient factors. This conceptual framework is modeled after the modified social-ecological model by Reifsnider and colleagues,[48] based on Bronfenbrenner's social-ecological model.

of diversity in the workforce has not been investigated. A decade ago, the pediatric rheumatology workforce was made up of greater than 90% white providers.[49] A recent study of subspecialist trainees in internal medicine over the past 10 years showed that rheumatology lagged behind other subspecialties in recruiting residents from race/ethnicities that were underrepresented in medicine.[50] Changes in the pediatric rheumatology workforce over the past decade have yet to be described.

Building diverse provider workforces regarding gender, race/ethnicity, and other sociodemographics is essential to address health disparities.[51] Severe mismatches in provider/patient sociodemographics may challenge the ability to give culturally competent care. Patient comfort and language preferences are also influenced by the presence or lack of diversity within the workforce; barriers to these can impede quality of care.

ADDRESSING DISPARITIES

Evidence-based approaches to address disparities in cSLE will rely not only on research that defines disparities but also on studies that test interventions (a) for how effective they are in at-risk populations and (b) so that these interventions not only improve outcomes but also close gaps in heath inequity (**Fig. 2**). Developing effective and appropriate interventions for at-risk populations requires partnerships with community members and other stakeholders to lead to change and improved care.

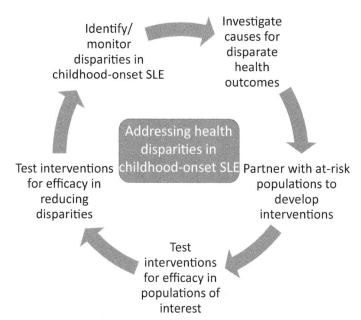

Fig. 2. Addressing health disparities in cSLE. A proposed iterative framework to address health disparities through evidence-based methods. This is modified from a conceptual framework developed by Rashid and colleagues.[56]

Some of this community-partnership work is underway. For example, to address presumed disparities in resources, access, and care to black and Latino communities, an educational intervention was developed to improve knowledge of SLE in reproductive health care providers from minority communities in New York with large black and Latino populations. A pilot of the intervention among reproductive health care providers showed improvement in self-reported knowledge and comfort in counseling adolescents and young women with SLE.[52]

SUMMARY

In this review of the literature on health disparities in cSLE, the authors found that there were disparities in prevalence, disease severity, morbidity, and mortality across race/ethnicity. Health care quality is adversely impacted by poverty and inaccessibility to pediatric rheumatologists on a regional level. Because of significant gaps in the literature, less is known about the contribution of income and other socioeconomic markers of disadvantage to outcomes of care.

Paralleling observations that have been noted in adult SLE literature,[53,54] black children with cSLE are at particularly high risk of poor outcomes and high morbidity. These disparities have been most well defined with regards to the risk of ESRD from LN, disparities in transplant rates, and mortality. The presence of these disparities in the pediatric population indicates that implementations only in older SLE patients may be missing the mark to effect change in adult patients with cSLE; earlier interventions in children with cSLE may bring about more equitable health outcomes among the black SLE patient population.

Few studies in cSLE have examined poverty and its impact on care and outcomes. Fewer studies have examined interactions between income and race/ethnicity. Some populations remain largely invisible in the literature. In literature from US centers, characterization of disease severity, care, and outcomes among Native American children with cSLE is largely absent, despite evidence that this may be a population at particular risk for both developing SLE and for being underserved specifically with regards to resources in pediatric rheumatologists and socially disadvantaged.

Authors of the reviewed studies have called for examining disparities in access to health care in youth with cSLE and the role that universal health care coverage may have to ameliorate health disparities for children with cSLE.[14] Although these are certainly warranted, the large studies of US Medicaid children[22,30] point to a problem that is more nuanced than simple health coverage.

Studies of health care quality and health care utilization among youth with cSLE are sparse. Work needs to be done with data that include at-risk youth from low-income backgrounds to understand and define potential disparities that have been observed in adult SLE populations.

Across the globe, observations, although preliminary, that youth with cSLE are more likely to come from socially disadvantaged and marginalized populations and that these populations are at particular risk for lower levels of care and worse outcomes, raise difficult questions about how damaging social structures, including systematic racism, may be affecting children at risk and with cSLE. Although these questions require further investigation, studies into understanding disparities need to be coupled with interventional studies looking at ways to ameliorate health inequities for children with cSLE.

This review was limited by the authors' very broad definition of health disparities, encompassing differences that are complex and multifactorial and that may include factors related to a wide variety of mechanisms of disease, system, and access differences in health care. More specific definitions of health disparities have been introduced to pinpoint inequities in care that are not accounted for by differences in access, preference, and need, including the definition used by the Institute of Medicine.[55] Few studies were designed to examine disparities in race/ethnicity while accounting for health care access and/or disease severity.

To better understand specific drivers for disparate outcomes among youth with SLE and adults with cSLE, future studies will have to leverage large disease registries that can account for multiple measures of access to care, race/ethnicity, income, and other measures of socioeconomic disadvantage.

DISCLOSURE

Funder: The Hospital for Sick Children, Ontario, Canada.

REFERENCES

1. Livingston B, Bonner A, Pope J. Differences in clinical manifestations between childhood-onset lupus and adult-onset lupus: a meta-analysis. Lupus 2011;20: 1345–55.

2. Sule S, Fivush B, Neu A, et al. Increased risk of death in pediatric and adult patients with ESRD secondary to lupus. Pediatr Nephrol 2011;26:93–8.

3. Kamphuis S, Silverman ED. Prevalence and burden of pediatric-onset systemic lupus erythematosus. Nat Rev Rheumatol 2010;6:538–46.

4. Knight AM, Weiss PF, Morales KH, et al. National trends in pediatric systemic lupus erythematosus hospitalization in the United States: 2000-2009. J Rheumatol 2014;41:539–46.

5. Hiraki LT, Feldman CH, Liu J, et al. Prevalence, incidence, and demographics of systemic lupus erythematosus and lupus nephritis from 2000 to 2004 among children in the US Medicaid beneficiary population. Arthritis Rheum 2012;64: 2669–76.

6. Mauldin J, Cameron HD, Jeanotte D, et al. Chronic arthritis in children and adolescents in two Indian health service user populations. BMC Musculoskelet Disord 2004;5:30.

7. Huang JL, Yao TC, See LC. Prevalence of pediatric systemic lupus erythematosus and juvenile chronic arthritis in a Chinese population: a nation-wide prospective population-based study in Taiwan. Clin Exp Rheumatol 2004;22:776–80.

8. Tucker LB, Uribe AG, Fernandez M, et al. Adolescent onset of lupus results in more aggressive disease and worse outcomes: results of a nested matched case-control study within Lumina, a multiethnic US cohort (Lumina LVII). Lupus 2008;17:314–22.

9. US Department of Health and Human Services. The Secretary's Advisory Committee on National Health Promotion and Disease Prevention Objectives for 2020. Phase I report: recommendations for the framework and format of healthy people 2020. Available at: https://www.healthypeople.gov/sites/default/files/PhaseI_0.pdf. Accessed January 23, 2020.

10. Houghton KM, Page J, Cabral DA, et al. Systemic lupus erythematosus in the pediatric North American Native population of British Columbia. J Rheumatol 2006; 33:161–3.

11. Huemer C, Huemer M, Dorner T, et al. Incidence of pediatric rheumatic diseases in a regional population in Austria. J Rheumatol 2001;28:2116–9.

12. Kaipiainen-Seppanen O, Savolainen A. Incidence of chronic juvenile rheumatic diseases in Finland during 1980-1990. Clin Exp Rheumatol 1996;14:441–4.

13. Denardo BA, Tucker LB, Miller LC, et al. Demography of a regional pediatric rheumatology patient population. Affiliated children's arthritis centers of New England. J Rheumatol 1994;21:1553–61.

14. Hiraki LT, Benseler SM, Tyrrell PN, et al. Ethnic differences in pediatric systemic lupus erythematosus. J Rheumatol 2009;36:2539–46.

15. Concannon A, Rudge S, Yan J, et al. The incidence, diagnostic clinical manifestations and severity of juvenile systemic lupus erythematosus in New Zealand Maori and Pacific Island children: the Starship Experience (2000-2010). Lupus 2013;22:1156–61.

16. Mackie FE, Kainer G, Adib N, et al. The national incidence and clinical picture of SLE in children in Australia - a report from the Australian Paediatric Surveillance Unit. Lupus 2015;24:66–73.

17. Sawhney S, Magalhães CS. Paediatric rheumatology–a global perspective. Best Pract Res Clin Rheumatol 2006;20(2):201–21.

18. Lewandowski LB, Watt MH, Schanberg LE, et al. Missed opportunities for timely diagnosis of pediatric lupus in South Africa: a qualitative study. Pediatr Rheumatol Online J 2017;15:14.

19. Tucker LB, Menon S, Schaller JG, et al. Adult- and childhood-onset systemic lupus erythematosus: a comparison of onset, clinical features, serology, and outcome. Br J Rheumatol 1995;34:866–72.

20. Smith EMD, Yin P, Jorgensen AL, et al. Clinical predictors of active LN development in children - evidence from the UK JSLE cohort study. Lupus 2018;27: 2020–8.

21. Lewandowski LB, Schanberg LE, Thielman N, et al. Severe disease presentation and poor outcomes among pediatric systemic lupus erythematosus patients in South Africa. Lupus 2017;26:186–94.

22. Knight AM, Xie M, Mandell DS. Disparities in psychiatric diagnosis and treatment for youth with systemic lupus erythematosus: analysis of a national US Medicaid sample. J Rheumatol 2016;43:1427–33.

23. Boneparth A, Ilowite NT, Investigators CR. Comparison of renal response parameters for juvenile membranous plus proliferative lupus nephritis versus isolated proliferative lupus nephritis: a cross-sectional analysis of the CARRA Registry. Lupus 2014;23:898–904.

24. Tan JH, Hoh SF, Win MT, et al. Childhood-onset systemic lupus erythematosus in Singapore: clinical phenotypes, disease activity, damage, and autoantibody profiles. Lupus 2015;24:998–1005.

25. Balkaran BN, Roberts LA, Ramcharan J. Systemic lupus erythematosus in Trinidadian children. Ann Trop Paediatr 2004;24:241–4.

26. Bakr A. Epidemiology treatment and outcome of childhood systemic lupus erythematosus in Egypt. Pediatr Nephrol 2005;20:1081–6.

27. Gunal N, Kara N, Akkok N, et al. Cardiac abnormalities in children with systemic lupus erythematosus. Turk J Pediatr 2003;45:301–5.

28. Sibbitt WL Jr, Brandt JR, Johnson CR, et al. The incidence and prevalence of neuropsychiatric syndromes in pediatric onset systemic lupus erythematosus. J Rheumatol 2002;29:1536–42.

29. Chang JC, Xiao R, Mercer-Rosa L, et al. Child-onset systemic lupus erythematosus is associated with a higher incidence of myopericardial manifestations compared to adult-onset disease. Lupus 2018;27:2146–54.

30. Harrison MJ, Zuhlke LJ, Lewandowski LB, et al. Pediatric systemic lupus erythematosus patients in South Africa have high prevalence and severity of cardiac and vascular manifestations. Pediatr Rheumatol Online J 2019;17:76.

31. Hiraki LT, Lu B, Alexander SR, et al. End-stage renal disease due to lupus nephritis among children in the US, 1995-2006. Arthritis Rheum 2011;63: 1988–97.

32. Costenbader KH, Desai A, Alarcon GS, et al. Trends in the incidence, demographics, and outcomes of end-stage renal disease due to lupus nephritis in the US from 1995 to 2006. Arthritis Rheum 2011;63:1681–8.

33. Lim LSHB S, Tyrrell P, Charron M. Osteopenia and osteoporosis already present in newly diagnosed juvenile systemic lupus erythematosus patients. J Rheumatol 2009;36:2586.

34. Miettunen PM, Ortiz-Alvarez O, Petty RE, et al. Gender and ethnic origin have no effect on longterm outcome of childhood-onset systemic lupus erythematosus. J Rheumatol 2004;31:1650–4.

35. Ravelli A, Duarte-Salazar C, Buratti S, et al. Assessment of damage in juvenile-onset systemic lupus erythematosus: a multicenter cohort study. Arthritis Rheum 2003;49:501–7.

36. Hersh AO, Case SM, Son MB, et al. Predictors of disability in a childhood-onset systemic lupus erythematosus cohort: results from the CARRA Legacy Registry. Lupus 2018;27:494–500.

37. Knight A, Weiss P, Morales K, et al. Depression and anxiety and their association with healthcare utilization in pediatric lupus and mixed connective tissue disease patients: a cross-sectional study. Pediatr Rheumatol Online J 2014;12:42.
38. Davis AM, Graham TB, Zhu Y, et al. Depression and medication nonadherence in childhood-onset systemic lupus erythematosus. Lupus 2018;27:1532–41.
39. Mina R, Klein-Gitelman MS, Nelson S, et al. Effects of obesity on health-related quality of life in juvenile-onset systemic lupus erythematosus. Lupus 2015;24: 191–7.
40. Moorthy LN, Baldino ME, Kurra V, et al. Relationship between health-related quality of life, disease activity and disease damage in a prospective international multicenter cohort of childhood onset systemic lupus erythematosus patients. Lupus 2017;26:255–65.
41. Levy DM, Peschken CA, Tucker LB, et al. Association of health-related quality of life in childhood-onset systemic lupus erythematosus with ethnicity: results from a multiethnic multicenter Canadian cohort. Arthritis Care Res (Hoboken) 2014;66: 1767–74.
42. Yazdany J, Trupin L, Tonner C, et al. Quality of care in systemic lupus erythematosus: application of quality measures to understand gaps in care. J Gen Intern Med 2012;27:1326–33.
43. Knight A, Weiss P, Morales K, et al. Epidemiology of the US national burden of pediatric lupus hospitalization from 2000-2009. Arthritis Rheumatol 2012;64: S403–4.
44. Chang JC, Knight AM, Lawson EF. Patterns of health care utilization and medication adherence among youth with systemic lupus erythematosus during transfer from pediatric to adult care. J Rheumatol 2020. jrheum.191029. [Online ahead of print].
45. Son MB, Sergeyenko Y, Guan H, et al. Disease activity and transition outcomes in a childhood-onset systemic lupus erythematosus cohort. Lupus 2016;25:1431–9.
46. Javalkar K, Johnson M, Kshirsagar AV, et al. Ecological factors predict transition readiness/self-management in youth with chronic conditions. J Adolesc Health 2016;58:40–6.
47. Rubinstein TB, Mowrey WB, Ilowite NT, et al. Childhood Arthritis and Rheumatology Research Alliance Investigators. Delays to care in pediatric lupus patients: data from the Childhood Arthritis and Rheumatology Research Alliance Legacy Registry. Arthritis Care Res (Hoboken) 2018;70:420–7.
48. Reifsnider E, Gallagher M, Forgione B. Using ecological models in research on health disparities. J Prof Nurs 2005;21:216–22.
49. Henrickson M. Policy challenges for the pediatric rheumatology workforce: part II. Health care system delivery and workforce supply. Pediatr Rheumatol Online J 2011;9:24.
50. Santhosh L, Babik JM. Trends in racial and ethnic diversity in internal medicine subspecialty fellowships from 2006 to 2018. JAMA Netw Open 2020;3:e1920482.
51. Jackson CS, Gracia JN. Addressing health and health-care disparities: the role of a diverse workforce and the social determinants of health. Public Health Rep 2014;129(Suppl 2):57–61.
52. Rose JA, Pichardo DM, Richey MC, et al. Lupus and reproductive health considerations: a pilot training for reproductive health care providers serving teens and young adults. Arthritis Rheum 2013;65:S389 [abstract].
53. Sexton DJ, Reule S, Solid C, et al. ESRD from lupus nephritis in the United States, 1995-2010. Clin J Am Soc Nephrol 2015;10:251–9.

54. Cooper GS, Treadwell EL, St Clair EW, et al. Sociodemographic associations with early disease damage in patients with systemic lupus erythematosus. Arthritis Rheum 2007;57:993–9.

55. Institute of Medicine. Unequal treatment: confronting racial and ethnic disparities in health care. Washington (DC): National Academy Press; 2002.

56. Rashid JR, Spengler RF, Wagner RM, et al. Eliminating health disparities through transdisciplinary research, cross-agency collaboration, and public participation. Am J Public Health 2009;99:1955–61.

Health Disparities in Systemic Lupus Erythematosus

Christine A. Peschken, MD, MSc, FRCPC

KEYWORDS

• Systemic lupus erythematosus • Health disparities • Social determinants of health

KEY POINTS

- In systemic lupus erythematosus (SLE), increased incidence and prevalence, more severe disease, and worse outcomes are well described in nonwhite ethnicities.
- Low adherence to lupus medications is common and relates to mistrust, cultural attitudes to health and disease, and poor patient-provider communication.
- Poverty significantly affects damage accrual and mortality for patients with SLE; recent evidence suggests the mechanism may be though chronic socioeconomic stressors.
- Health care access is adversely influenced by racism and geography, and contributes to poor adherence and increased damage and mortality. Ethnic minorities and the poor may be at higher risk for hazardous environmental exposures contributing to the burden of SLE in these populations.
- Epigenetic changes may provide the link between social adversity and poor lupus outcomes, and may provide a pathway to a better understanding of SLE pathogenesis and personalized treatment approaches.

INTRODUCTION

Health disparities have been defined as differences in the incidence, prevalence, outcomes, and burden of diseases and other adverse health conditions that exist among different population groups, and, most importantly, these differences are considered unnecessary and avoidable.[1] The study of health disparities has been recognized as a priority by multiple countries, groups, and government bodies.[2,3] Systemic lupus erythematosus (SLE) in many ways can be seen to epitomize health disparities. SLE is more prevalent among women and in ethnic minority and Indigenous populations. Outcomes are also worse in these groups, as well as in people of lower socioeconomic status. The many factors that influence outcomes in SLE are complex, overlapping, and closely associated with each other. Ethnic differences in incidence, prevalence,

Rady Faculty of Health Sciences, University of Manitoba, RR149 Arthritis Centre, 800 Sherbrook Street, Winnipeg, Manitoba R3A1M4, Canada
E-mail address: christine.peschken@umanitoba.ca

Rheum Dis Clin N Am 46 (2020) 673–683
https://doi.org/10.1016/j.rdc.2020.07.010
0889-857X/20/© 2020 Elsevier Inc. All rights reserved.

and outcomes are the most prominent and best-described disparity in SLE; herein is a brief review of disparities closely associated with ethnicity. Particular emphasis is placed on Indigenous North Americans with SLE because there is a paucity of data for this group.

INCIDENCE, PREVALENCE, AND MORTALITY

Differences in incidence and prevalence rates between ethnic groups have been clearly documented over many years.[4] The US Centers for Disease Control and Prevention (CDC) has funded surveillance programs as part of a national public health agenda for lupus to prioritize a coordinated and multifaceted public health approach to lupus[5] and have recently shown that the prevalence of SLE in the United States was highest among American Indian/Alaskan native (Indigenous North American) women (271; 95% confidence interval [CI], 238, 307) and black women (230.9; 95% CI, 178.2, 299.2), followed by Hispanic women (120.7; 95% CI, 84.0, 173.4) compared with white women and Asian Pacific Islander women, both of whom had a prevalence about 84 per 100,000.[6] This work echoes multiple previous publications documenting the higher incidence and prevalence rates in essentially all nonwhite ethnic/racial groups.[7]

Patients with SLE have long been known to have excess mortality, with rates of 2 to 5 times that of the general population, confirmed in a recent meta-analysis including more than 26,000 patients with SLE.[8] Jorge and colleagues[9] showed that this mortality gap has not improved in recent decades. Ethnic disparities in mortality from lupus are stark. Yen and colleagues,[10] using the CDC's national vital statistics system mortality database, showed that SLE was among the leading causes of death in young women. Overall, SLE was in the top 20 leading causes of death for all women and ranked 10th in women aged 15 to 24 years. However, SLE was the fifth leading cause among black and Hispanic women aged 15 to 24 years after excluding injury as a cause of death from the analysis. In another study of more than 40,000 patients with prevalent SLE, Indigenous North American and black patients had the highest mortalities, with lower risks among Hispanic and Asian patients with SLE, after accounting for demographic and clinical factors.[11] Similarly, in a Canadian study, Indigenous North Americans had a 2-fold hazard ratio for mortality compared with white SLE patients, after adjustment for income, education, and rural residence.[12] Also striking in this study was the young age at death of Indigenous patients compared with white patients from the same center. Mean age at death was 50 years in Indigenous patients, compared with 64 years for white patients, translating into potential years of life lost for Indigenous patients of 6.5 per 1000 compared with 2.6 per 1000 in white patients.

RENAL OUTCOMES

Lupus nephritis remains one of the most serious complications of SLE; disparities in renal outcomes mirror disparities in incidence, prevalence, and mortality. The LUMINA (Lupus in Minorities, Nature vs Nurture) study showed higher frequency of lupus nephritis in US African American and Hispanic patients[13] compared with white patients. In a larger Medicaid study of more than 34,000 patients with SLE, all nonwhite patients, including African American, Asian, Hispanic, and Indigenous North American, had a higher prevalence of lupus nephritis.[14] Similarly, in the United Kingdom, Chinese, Afro-Caribbean and Indo-Asian patients with SLE had more frequent nephritis,[15] and, in Canadian cohorts, Asian, black, and Indigenous Canadian patients with SLE had more frequent nephritis.[12,16,17] In addition to more frequent development of nephritis, nonwhite patients develop nephritis earlier in their disease course compared with white patients.[13,18] Progression to end-stage renal disease (ESRD) also differs between ethnicities: higher rates of progression to ESRD caused by SLE were described in African American, Asian, and Indigenous North American patients, with no changes in outcomes over the last decade.[19] Higher rates of renal damage/ESRD in nonwhite patients were also reported in Canadian and European cohorts.[17,20,21] In our single-center cohort, both Asian and Indigenous North American patients with SLE had a higher likelihood of developing nephritis, and a 5-fold risk of ESRD compared with white patients (**Fig. 1**). After adjustment for income, education, age, damage, and additional disease manifestations, the hazard ratio for ESRD was more than 6-fold for Asian and Indigenous patients with lupus nephritis compared with white patients with lupus nephritis.

Ward[22] showed that ESRD caused by lupus nephritis was increased in areas with higher rates of hospitalizations for ambulatory care–sensitive conditions, and also in areas with Medicaid insurance for a higher proportion of hospitalizations, suggesting insufficient coverage to access appropriate and/or quality care. Nonwhite ethnicity and lack of private insurance were associated with suboptimal quality of care for ESRD care in another large US study.[23]

Mortality in patients with lupus nephritis is more complex. Among more than 8000 Medicaid patients with lupus nephritis, Indigenous North American and black patients had higher mortality compared with white patients, whereas Asian and Hispanic patients with lupus nephritis had a lower mortality after adjustment for comorbidities and sociodemographic factors.[11] Although lupus nephritis as well as progression to ESRD was more frequent in Asian compared with Indigenous and white patients (see **Fig. 1**), preliminary Canadian data showed higher mortality in Indigenous North American patients with lupus nephritis and ESRD compared with Asian and white patients.[21] US Asian and Hispanic patients with ESRD caused by lupus nephritis also had lower mortality compared with white and African American patients.[24] Higher mortality in African Americans with ESRD caused by lupus has been found in several studies.[25,26] Overall improvement in mortality for patients with SLE with ESRD was recently shown, but the gap between white people and African Americans remained.[27]

436/920 patients developed lupus nephritis over their disease course (47%)
46/436 patients with lupus nephritis progressed to end-stage renal disease (11%)

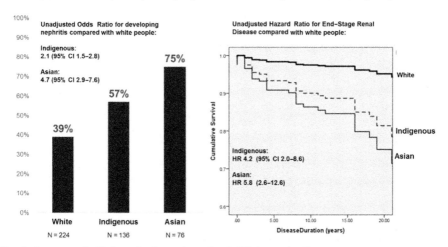

Fig. 1. Lupus nephritis in a single-center cohort. HR, hazard ratio.

ADHERENCE

Medication adherence is recognized as an important issue worldwide in the management of chronic disease,[28] including lupus.[29] Poor adherence to prescribed medications is associated with poor overall outcomes, disease progression, and an estimated burden of billions of dollars per year in avoidable direct health care costs.[28,30] Although low adherence is widespread, the frequently asymptomatic nature of lupus flares may contribute to low adherence,[31] particularly in lupus nephritis.[32,33] Almost 30 years ago, Petri and colleagues[34] reported that poor outcomes in black patients with SLE were related to low adherence rather than race or socioeconomic status. Since then, multiple studies have documented lower adherence in nonwhite patients.[11,31,35-39] This lower adherence includes adherence to hydroxychloroquine, recognized as important background therapy in SLE, which is reportedly lower in ethnic minorities,[40] and adherence to common immunosuppressive medications for SLE.[41]

Note that adherence to treatment implies that agreement to a care plan has initially been established between the patient and the health care provider. There is ample evidence that this initial agreement is often lacking, particularly in ethnic minorities, thus it perhaps should not be surprising that these groups have low overall rates of adherence. Adherence depends heavily on trust in the provider and the health care system, and on the patient-physician relationship and communication.[28,31] There is often a high degree of mistrust among ethnic minorities toward health care providers, based on a combination of past history of mistreatment and current perceived discrimination.[31,42] Experiences of discrimination in health care are pervasive among ethnic minorities and are associated with poor health care behaviors, including low adherence.[43] Cultural differences may also affect adherence; ethnic minorities may view health, illness, and medication through a different cultural lens.[28,31,44-46] These differences must be acknowledged and incorporated into health education and doctor-patient communication to improve adherence.

POVERTY

The association between poverty and poor disease outcomes has been well established in lupus[47-49]; income levels and ethnicity frequently cluster together. In the LUMINA cohort, investigators showed that poverty, not ethnicity, predicted increased mortality in SLE, with the effect of ethnicity only becoming evident in multivariate models with poverty removed.[50] Cooper and colleagues[51] found ethnicity and low income to be independently associated with poor outcomes in terms of increased damage. More recently, several studies have shown that neighborhood poverty (residing in an area with high poverty rates) contributes to damage and mortality independently of individual income level, although living in an area with a high proportion of people living in poverty accentuated the effect of individual low income on damage accrual.[52] Yelin and colleagues,[47] in the Lupus Outcomes Study, showed that the impact of poverty on mortality was through increased damage accrual. Importantly, there was a rapid normalization of damage accrual among patients with SLE who exited poverty.[52] Higher levels of perceived stress have been shown to be a likely mechanism for the effect of poverty on damage accrual. In a qualitative analysis, chronic socioeconomic stressors such as food insecurity, housing inability, and medical care insecurity, combined with exposure to crime, significantly affected patients with SLE. These stressors were described as requiring all of the patients' focus and attention, leaving SLE symptoms neglected until unavoidable.[53] There is increasing evidence of the impact of poverty on such decision making. Some researchers refer to bandwidth: the brain's ability to perform basic functions required for decision making. When taxed by such stressors as those discussed earlier, less bandwidth is available, leading to potentially undesirable health-related choices and behaviors.[54]

HEALTH CARE ACCESS

Access to health care is strongly linked to outcome of SLE, with clear demonstrations of increased damage accrual and increased mortality in low-income patients with lupus with less access. However, access to care goes beyond the merely financial and includes disparities in patient-physician communication[55] and concerns about racism and cultural safety within health care.[56–58]Experiences of racism and poor communication are deterrents to seeking health care, even when available. This tendency has been clearly shown for both Canadian and American Indigenous patients, who frequently characterize health care interactions as negative, with associated reluctance to seek care.[58–60]

Access to health care is also influenced by geography. In a nationwide US survey, rural residents and African Americans had a greater travel burden when seeking medical care.[61] In a South Carolina study, increased travel burden translated into more missed appointments and missed medications.[62] Mean travel time to lupus-associated medical care was approximately 57 minutes (ranging from 4 to 150 minutes), and the average distance to rheumatologists was approximately 85 km (53 miles). In Canada, Indigenous patients frequently live in remote communities. Indigenous people experience specific challenges accessing health care across all geographic regions, but challenges are greatest in rural and remote communities.[63] In our region, more than half of Indigenous patients lived greater than 160 km (100 miles) away, with 30% living more than 500 km (300 miles) from rheumatology care, frequently without road access. We showed that distance from rheumatology care had a significant impact on mortality (**Fig. 2**). Low income and educational attainment both increased mortality, independently of ethnicity (see **Fig. 2**). Indigenous patients were overrepresented in the low-income, low-education, and remote-from-care groups, showing the overlapping nature of these factors. In a Cox proportional hazards model, after adjusting for gender, onset age, disease duration and severity, and damage, as well as income and education, Indigenous ethnicity remained an independent risk for mortality (hazard ratio, 1.8; 95% CI, 1.1–3.0).[12]

ENVIRONMENTAL EXPOSURES

Environmental exposures are increasingly recognized as contributing to both the onset and subsequent disease course of SLE. There is robust evidence that cigarette smoking is associated with both the onset of SLE and a more severe disease course.[64] Here too, disparities may play a role: tobacco use, although reduced overall, has shifted from a mainstream behavior to a behavior that is mainly is concentrated among marginalized populations.[65] Maynard and colleagues[66] found that, in both white people and African Americans with SLE, individuals in the lowest income category had the highest frequency of current or past smoking; similarly, the lowest education category was also associated with the highest frequency of smoking. Secondhand smoke exposure in nonsmokers has also been shown to be higher in nonwhite people and in the poor.[67] Silica exposure has also been clearly shown to contribute to the development of SLE, and there is emerging evidence that exposure to air pollution, solvents, heavy metals, and pesticides may contribute to lupus development and disease activity.[68–71] These exposures vary by occupation and neighborhood residence. Thus, ethnic minorities and the poor are more likely to be exposed to

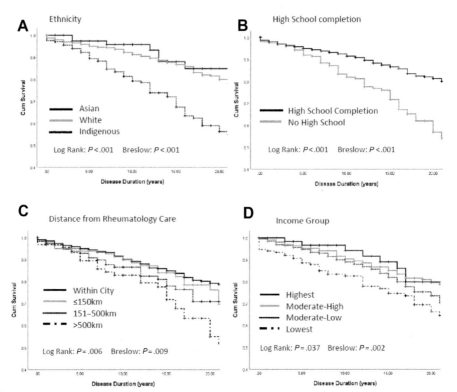

Fig. 2. Kaplan-Meier survival curves factors influencing mortality in Systemic lupus erythematosus patients from a single-center cohort. (*A*) Ethnicity. (*B*) High School Completion. (*C*) Distance from rheumatology care. (*D*) Household income.

hazardous substances in their neighborhoods and harmful working environments through low-wage jobs, further contributing to poor health outcomes.[72]

EPIGENETIC CHANGES

SLE is known to be caused by interactions between susceptibility genes and environmental factors. Distinct differences in disease-susceptibility genetic variants between ethnic groups have been described,[73,74] but, overall, genetic studies have failed to adequately explain the variable susceptibility, disease course, and outcomes of SLE across diverse populations.[75,76] Epigenetic mechanisms may provide that link.[77] In a study to address the clinical heterogeneity of SLE, Lanata and colleagues[78] identified clustering of severe disease phenotypes with nonwhite ethnicity, and also methylation differences between the clinical clusters, possibly reflecting environmental exposures that affect races differentially. Although studies linking specific adverse experiences or behaviors to epigenetic changes in SLE are lacking, mounting evidence across many diseases suggests that epigenetic mechanisms may provide a causal link between social adversity and health disparity.[79] Further epigenetic research promises to shed light on the molecular pathways through which such exposures are translated into quantifiable increased risk of SLE and poor SLE outcomes.[80]

SUMMARY

As clinicians look with optimism and hope toward recently approved and "pipeline" drugs, they should keep in mind the ample evidence showing that improving the environments in which patients live, work, and receive care, from health care systems and neighborhoods, to environmental exposures, to experiences of discrimination, would have a far greater impact on SLE outcomes than new medications. Without attention to these modifiable disparities, outcomes for vulnerable patients with SLE will continue to lag.

FUNDING ACKNOWLEDGEMENTS

Dr. Peschken has received funding for her research from Lupus Canada and the Lupus Society of Manitoba.

REFERENCES

1. Whitehead M. The concepts and principles of equity and health. Int J Health Serv 1992;22(3):429–45.
2. Braveman P. What are health disparities and health equity? We need to be clear. Public Health Rep 2014;129(Suppl 2):5–8.
3. Public Health Agency of Canada. (2018). Key Health Inequalities in Canada: A National Portrait. Ottawa: Author https://www.canada.ca/content/dam/phac-aspc/documents/services/publications/science-research/key-health-inequalities-canada-national-portrait-executive-summary/key_health_inequalities_full_report-eng.pdf
4. Rees F, Doherty M, Grainge MJ, et al. The worldwide incidence and prevalence of systemic lupus erythematosus: a systematic review of epidemiological studies. Rheumatology (Oxford) 2017;56(11):1945–61.
5. National Association of Chronic Disease Directors and the Lupus Foundation of America. (2015). National public health agenda for lupus. Available at: https://b.3cdn.net/lupus/8085bc0a72575355b2_lfm6zqgst.pdf
6. Somers E, Wang L, McCune W, et al. Prevalence of systemic lupus erythematosus in the united states: preliminary estimates from a meta-analysis of the centers for disease control and prevention lupus registries [abstract]. Arthritis Rheumatol 2019;71(suppl 10). Available at: https://acrabstracts.org/abstract/prevalence-of-systemic-lupus-erythematosus-in-the-united-states-preliminary-estimates-from-a-meta-analysis-of-the-centers-for-disease-control-and-prevention-lupus-registries/.
7. Lewis MJ, Jawad AS. The effect of ethnicity and genetic ancestry on the epidemiology, clinical features and outcome of systemic lupus erythematosus. Rheumatology (Oxford) 2017;56(suppl_1):i67–77.
8. Lee YH, Choi SJ, Ji JD, et al. Overall and cause-specific mortality in systemic lupus erythematosus: an updated meta-analysis. Lupus 2016;25(7):727–34.
9. Jorge AM, Lu N, Zhang Y, et al. Unchanging premature mortality trends in systemic lupus erythematosus: a general population-based study (1999-2014). Rheumatology (Oxford) 2018;57(2):337–44.
10. Yen EY, Singh RR. Brief report: lupus-an unrecognized leading cause of death in young females: a population-based study using nationwide death certificates, 2000-2015. Arthritis Rheumatol 2018;70(8):1251–5.
11. Gomez-Puerta JA, Barbhaiya M, Guan H, et al. Racial/Ethnic variation in all-cause mortality among United States medicaid recipients with systemic lupus erythematosus: a Hispanic and asian paradox. Arthritis Rheumatol 2015;67(3):752–60.
12. Puar RHC, Robinson D, Dhindsa N, El-Gabalawy H, Peschken C. High mortality in vulnerable Canadians with systemic Lupus erythematosus. (abstract) J Rheumatol 2015;42:1267. https://doi.org/10.3899/jrheum.150322.

13. Burgos PI, McGwin G Jr, Pons-Estel GJ, et al. US patients of Hispanic and African ancestry develop lupus nephritis early in the disease course: data from LUMINA, a multiethnic US cohort (LUMINA LXXIV). Ann Rheum Dis 2011;70(2):393–4.

14. Feldman CH, Hiraki LT, Liu J, et al. Epidemiology and sociodemographics of systemic lupus erythematosus and lupus nephritis among US adults with Medicaid coverage, 2000-2004. Arthritis Rheum 2013;65(3):753–63.

15. Patel M, Clarke AM, Bruce IN, et al. The prevalence and incidence of biopsy-proven lupus nephritis in the UK: Evidence of an ethnic gradient. Arthritis Rheum 2006;54(9):2963–9.

16. Peschken CA, Katz SJ, Silverman E, et al. The 1000 Canadian faces of lupus: determinants of disease outcome in a large multiethnic cohort. J Rheumatol 2009; 36(6):1200–8.

17. Johnson SR, Urowitz MB, Ibanez D, et al. Ethnic variation in disease patterns and health outcomes in systemic lupus erythematosus. J Rheumatol 2006;33(10): 1990–5.

18. Pons-Estel GJ, Alarcon GS, Burgos PI, et al. Mestizos with systemic lupus erythematosus develop renal disease early while antimalarials retard its appearance: data from a Latin American cohort. Lupus 2013;22(9):899–907.

19. Costenbader KH, Desai A, Alarcon GS, et al. Trends in the incidence, demographics, and outcomes of end-stage renal disease due to lupus nephritis in the US from 1995 to 2006. Arthritis Rheum 2011;63(6):1681–8.

20. Cervera R, Doria A, Amoura Z, et al. Patterns of systemic lupus erythematosus expression in Europe. Autoimmun Rev 2014;13(6):621–9.

21. Peschken C, Gole R, Hitchon C, et al. Outcomes of lupus nephritis in vulnerable populations. Arthritis Rheumatol 2017;69(suppl 10) [abstract]. Available at: https://acrabstracts.org/abstract/outcomes-of-lupus-nephritis-in-vulnerable-populations/.

22. Ward MM. Access to care and the incidence of endstage renal disease due to systemic lupus erythematosus. J Rheumatol 2010;37(6):1158–63.

23. Plantinga LC, Drenkard C, Patzer RE, et al. Sociodemographic and geographic predictors of quality of care in United States patients with end-stage renal disease due to lupus nephritis. Arthritis Rheumatol 2015;67(3):761–72.

24. Gomez-Puerta JA, Feldman CH, Alarcon GS, et al. Racial and ethnic differences in mortality and cardiovascular events among patients with end-stage renal disease due to lupus nephritis. Arthritis Care Res 2015;67(10):1453–62.

25. Nee R, Jindal RM, Little D, et al. Racial differences and income disparities are associated with poor outcomes in kidney transplant recipients with lupus nephritis. Transplantation 2013;95(12):1471–8.

26. Sule S, Fivush B, Neu A, et al. Increased risk of death in African American patients with end-stage renal disease secondary to lupus. Clin Kidney J 2014; 7(1):40–4.

27. Jorge A, Wallace ZS, Zhang Y, et al. All-cause and cause-specific mortality trends of end-stage renal disease due to lupus nephritis from 1995 to 2014. Arthritis Rheumatol 2019;71(3):403–10.

28. Brown MT, Bussell JK. Medication adherence: WHO cares? Mayo Clin Proc 2011; 86(4):304–14.

29. Costedoat-Chalumeau N, Pouchot J, Guettrot-Imbert G, et al. Adherence to treatment in systemic lupus erythematosus patients. Best Pract Res Clin Rheumatol 2013;27(3):329–40.

30. Costedoat-Chalumeau N, Tamirou F, Piette JC. Treatment adherence in systemic lupus erythematosus and rheumatoid arthritis: time to focus on this important issue. Rheumatology (Oxford) 2018;57(9):1507–9.

31. Brown MT, Bussell J, Dutta S, et al. Medication Adherence: Truth and Consequences. Am J Med Sci 2016;351(4):387–99.

32. Ali AY, Abdelaziz TS, Essameldin M. The prevalence and causes non-adherence to immunosuppressive medications in patients with Lupus nephritis flares. Curr Rheumatol Rev 2019. https://doi.org/10.2174/1573397115666190626111847.

33. Yo JH, Barbour TD, Nicholls K. Management of refractory lupus nephritis: challenges and solutions. Open Access Rheumatol 2019;11:179–88.

34. Petri M, Perez-Gutthann S, Longenecker JC, et al. Morbidity of systemic lupus erythematosus: role of race and socioeconomic status. Am J Med 1991;91(4):345–53.

35. Heidenreich PA. Patient adherence: the next frontier in quality improvement. Am J Med 2004;117(2):130–2.

36. Xie Z, St Clair P, Goldman DP, et al. Racial and ethnic disparities in medication adherence among privately insured patients in the United States. PLoS One 2019;14(2):e0212117.

37. Feldman CH, Costenbader KH, Solomon DH, et al. Area-Level Predictors of Medication Nonadherence Among US Medicaid Beneficiaries With Lupus: A Multilevel Study. Arthritis Care Res 2019;71(7):903–13.

38. Feldman CH, Yazdany J, Guan H, et al. Medication nonadherence is associated with increased subsequent acute care utilization among medicaid beneficiaries with systemic lupus erythematosus. Arthritis Care Res 2015;67(12):1712–21.

39. Hoi A. Asian lupus in a multi-ethnic society: what can be learnt? Int J Rheum Dis 2015;18(2):113–6.

40. Feldman CH, Collins J, Zhang Z, et al. Dynamic patterns and predictors of hydroxychloroquine nonadherence among Medicaid beneficiaries with systemic lupus erythematosus. Semin Arthritis Rheum 2018;48(2):205–13.

41. Feldman CH, Collins J, Zhang Z, et al. Azathioprine and mycophenolate mofetil adherence patterns and predictors among medicaid beneficiaries with systemic lupus erythematosus. Arthritis Care Res 2019;71(11):1419–24.

42. Muller E, Zill JM, Dirmaier J, et al. Assessment of trust in physician: a systematic review of measures. PLoS One 2014;9(9):e106844.

43. Williams DR, Lawrence JA, Davis BA, et al. Understanding how discrimination can affect health. Health Serv Res 2019;54(Suppl 2):1374–88.

44. Shahin W, Kennedy GA, Stupans I. The impact of personal and cultural beliefs on medication adherence of patients with chronic illnesses: a systematic review. Patient Prefer Adherence 2019;13:1019–35.

45. Jin L, Acharya L. Cultural beliefs underlying medication adherence in people of chinese descent in the United States. Health Commun 2016;31(5):513–21.

46. Bosworth HB, Granger BB, Mendys P, et al. Medication adherence: a call for action. Am Heart J 2011;162(3):412–24.

47. Yelin E, Yazdany J, Trupin L. Relationship between poverty and mortality in systemic lupus erythematosus. Arthritis Care Res 2018;70(7):1101–6.

48. Demas KL, Costenbader KH. Disparities in lupus care and outcomes. Curr Opin Rheumatol 2009;21(2):102–9.

49. Walsh SJ, Gilchrist A. Geographical clustering of mortality from systemic lupus erythematosus in the United States: contributions of poverty, Hispanic ethnicity and solar radiation. Lupus 2006;15(10):662–70.

50. Alarcon GS. Lessons from LUMINA: a multiethnic US cohort. Lupus 2008;17(11): 971–6.

51. Cooper GS, Treadwell EL, St Clair EW, et al. Sociodemographic associations with early disease damage in patients with systemic lupus erythematosus. Arthritis Rheum 2007;57(6):993–9.

52. Yelin E, Trupin L, Yazdany J. A prospective study of the impact of current poverty, history of poverty, and exiting poverty on accumulation of disease damage in systemic lupus erythematosus. Arthritis Rheumatol 2017;69(8):1612–22.

53. Yelin E, Trupin L, Bunde J, et al. Poverty, neighborhoods, persistent stress, and systemic lupus erythematosus outcomes: a qualitative study of the patients' perspective. Arthritis Care Res 2019;71(3):398–405.

54. Schilbach F, Schofield H, Mullainathan S. The psychological lives of the poor. Am Econ Rev 2016;106(5):435–40.

55. Yelin E, Yazdany J, Trupin L. Relationship between process of care and a subsequent increase in damage in systemic lupus erythematosus. Arthritis Care Res 2017;69(6):927–32.

56. McNally M, Martin D. First Nations, Inuit and Métis health: Considerations for Canadian health leaders in the wake of the Truth and Reconciliation Commission of Canada report. Healthc Manage Forum 2017;30(2):117–22.

57. Mehat P, Atiquzzaman M, Esdaile JM, et al. Medication nonadherence in systemic lupus erythematosus: a systematic review. Arthritis Care Res 2017; 69(11):1706–13.

58. Lavoie JG. Medicare and the care of First Nations, Métis and Inuit. Health Econ Policy Law 2018;13(3–4):280–98.

59. Twumasi AA, Shao A, Dunlop-Thomas C, et al. Health service utilization among African American women living with systemic lupus erythematosus: perceived impacts of a self-management intervention. Arthritis Res Ther 2019;21(1):155.

60. Chae DH, Martz CD, Fuller-Rowell TE, et al. Racial discrimination, disease activity, and organ damage: the black women's experiences living with lupus (BeWELL) Study. Am J Epidemiol 2019;188(8):1434–43.

61. Probst JC, Laditka SB, Wang JY, et al. Effects of residence and race on burden of travel for care: cross sectional analysis of the 2001 US National Household Travel Survey. BMC Health Serv Res 2007;7:40.

62. Williams EM, Ortiz K, Zhang J, et al. The systemic lupus erythematosus travel burden survey: baseline data among a South Carolina cohort. BMC Res Notes 2016;9:246.

63. National Collaborating Centre for Aboriginal health (NCCAH). Access to health services as a social determinants of first Nations, Inuit and Metis health. Prince George (BC): 2019. Available at: https://www.nccih.ca/docs/determinants/FS-AccessHealthServicesSDOH-2019-EN.pdf

64. Speyer CB, Costenbader KH. Cigarette smoking and the pathogenesis of systemic lupus erythematosus. Expert Rev Clin Immunol 2018;14(6):481–7.

65. Assari S, Bazargan M. Unequal effects of educational attainment on workplace exposure to second-hand smoke by race and ethnicity; minorities' diminished returns in the national health interview survey (NHIS). J Med Res Innov 2019;3(2). https://doi.org/10.32892/jmri.179.

66. Maynard JW, Fang H, Petri M. Low socioeconomic status is associated with cardiovascular risk factors and outcomes in systemic lupus erythematosus. J Rheumatol 2012;39(4):777–83.

67. Tsai J, Homa DM, Gentzke AS, et al. Exposure to Secondhand Smoke Among Nonsmokers - United States, 1988-2014. MMWR Morb Mortal Wkly Rep 2018; 67(48):1342–6.

68. Barbhaiya M, Costenbader KH. Environmental exposures and the development of systemic lupus erythematosus. Curr Opin Rheumatol 2016;28(5):497–505.

69. Carter EE, Barr SG, Clarke AE. The global burden of SLE: prevalence, health disparities and socioeconomic impact. Nat Rev Rheumatol 2016;12(10):605–20.

70. Cooper GS, Parks CG. Occupational and environmental exposures as risk factors for systemic lupus erythematosus. Curr Rheumatol Rep 2004;6(5):367–74.

71. Kamen DL. Environmental influences on systemic lupus erythematosus expression. Rheum Dis Clin North Am 2014;40(3):401–12, vii.

72. Kramer MR, Hogue CR. Is segregation bad for your health? Epidemiol Rev 2009; 31:178–94.

73. Hanscombe KB, Morris DL, Noble JA, et al. Genetic fine mapping of systemic lupus erythematosus MHC associations in Europeans and African Americans. Hum Mol Genet 2018;27(21):3813–24.

74. Langefeld CD, Ainsworth HC, Cunninghame Graham DS, et al. Transancestral mapping and genetic load in systemic lupus erythematosus. Nat Commun 2017;8:16021.

75. Leffers HCB, Lange T, Collins C, et al. The study of interactions between genome and exposome in the development of systemic lupus erythematosus. Autoimmun Rev 2019;18(4):382–92.

76. Gulati G, Brunner HI. Environmental triggers in systemic lupus erythematosus. Semin Arthritis Rheum 2018;47(5):710–7.

77. Long H, Yin H, Wang L, et al. The critical role of epigenetics in systemic lupus erythematosus and autoimmunity. J Autoimmun 2016;74:118–38.

78. Lanata CM, Paranjpe I, Nititham J, et al. A phenotypic and genomics approach in a multi-ethnic cohort to subtype systemic lupus erythematosus. Nat Commun 2019;10(1):3902.

79. Notterman DA, Mitchell C. Epigenetics and understanding the impact of social determinants of health. Pediatr Clin North Am 2015;62(5):1227–40.

80. Bowers ME, Yehuda R. Intergenerational transmission of stress in humans. Neuropsychopharmacology 2016;41(1):232–44.

Disparities in Rheumatoid Arthritis Care and Health Service Solutions to Equity

Cheryl Barnabe, MD, MSc, FRCPC[a,b],*

KEYWORDS

- Rheumatoid arthritis • Inequities • Access to care • Quality improvement
- Models of care

KEY POINTS

- Rheumatoid arthritis care access varies by rural and remote residence, race and ethnicity, and socioeconomic status, contributing to undesirable disease outcomes.
- Populations characterized by age, sex, race and ethnicity, sex, socioeconomic status, and location of residence experience substantial difficulties in accessing evidence-based rheumatoid arthritis treatment.
- Adherence to quality care indicators and patient experience in rheumatology care are important areas for research and action for resolving care gaps for populations at risk for inequities in rheumatoid arthritis outcomes.
- Promising health service interventions and therapeutic decision-making supports are potential solutions to better support optimal rheumatoid arthritis outcomes.

INTRODUCTION

Paradigm shifts in the recognition and treatment of rheumatoid arthritis (RA) have occurred over the past 2 decades, improving the frequency with which major treatment goals of remission and prevention of damage and disability are achieved.[1] Prioritization of assessment of suspected inflammatory arthritis within weeks of onset, coupled with frequent reassessment and aggressive adjustment of therapy to achieve objective determination of remission (treat-to-target) are widely accepted as standard of care and appear in major treatment guidelines[2,3] and as performance measures.[4] Implementation of models of care to support these tenets and thereby attain these standards in practice necessitates restructuring of systems and clinics. However, redesign and reconfiguration of systems of practice are largely oriented to meet needs

[a] Department of Medicine, Cumming School of Medicine, University of Calgary, 3330 Hospital Drive Northwest, Calgary, AB T2N 4N1, Canada; [b] Department of Community Health Sciences, Cumming School of Medicine, University of Calgary, 3330 Hospital Drive Northwest, Calgary, AB T2N 4N1, Canada
* Department of Medicine, Cumming School of Medicine, University of Calgary, 3330 Hospital Drive Northwest, Calgary, AB T2N 4N1, Canada.
E-mail address: ccbarnab@ucalgary.ca

Rheum Dis Clin N Am 46 (2020) 685–692
https://doi.org/10.1016/j.rdc.2020.07.005
rheumatic.theclinics.com
0889-857X/20/© 2020 The Author(s). Published by Elsevier Inc. This is an open access article under the CC BY-NC-ND license (http://creativecommons.org/licenses/by-nc-nd/4.0/).

of the population majority, introducing the possibility that intervention-generated in-equalities and equity harms[5] for those populations who were already at risk for ineq-uities in outcomes result and thus with unintended consequences of widening care gaps.

Conceptualization of which populations may be negatively affected by interventions is facilitated by using the PROGRESS Plus framework. PROGRESS Plus is an acronym identifying population groups at risk for inequities, which includes Place of residence; Race/ethnicity/culture/language; Occupation; Gender/sex; Religion; Edu-cation; Socioeconomic Status; and Social capital; and with Plus referring to personal characteristics associated with discrimination, features of relationships, and time-dependent relationships including transitions in care.[6,7] Athough summarizing outcome variations for each of these populations, as well as considering aspects of intersectionality (whereby patients experience exponential gaps by their membership in several populations experiencing disparities and inequities) is beyond the scope of this article, examples of described disparities in health services delivery, medication access, and quality of care considerations specific to RA care paradigms in the United States and Canada will be provided. Further, proposed models of care and treatment approaches that can better support optimal RA outcomes will be summarized.

DISPARITIES IN ACCESS TO HEALTH SERVICES

Geography introduces risk for inequities in health outcomes based on differences in physical environments and health care availability compared with urban populations, and this affects the ability to minimize time to diagnosis and provide frequent reas-sessment of disease activity. As an example of diagnostic delay introduced by geographic distance to rheumatology providers, in a Canadian study, remote distance (defined as residence >100 km to rheumatologist) was associated with a nearly 50% lower odds of being seen by a rheumatologist within 3 months of suspected diagnosis, even after adjustment for patient demographics, clinical factors, primary care physi-cian characteristics, provider continuity, and geographic characteristics.[8] Remote dis-tance from providers was also associated with an approximately 70% reduction in continuity in care in the first year of disease onset.[8] In a study of US-based Medicare patients older than 65 years of age, persons with the longest driving distances to rheu-matology providers had an approximately 30% decreased odds of receiving an RA diagnosis compared with those located nearest to rheumatology care.[9]

Socioeconomic status is also a determinant of health service access for RA care. Although limited by study design requiring self-report of RA status, a study of patients aged 18 to 64 years found that uninsured and Medicaid patients in the United States were 17% and 13% less likely to visit a rheumatologist, respectively.[10]

Decreased health service access for diagnosis and continuing care may result in accumulation of RA damage, leading to surgical needs. In an American Medicare cohort, rural residents with RA had 30% higher odds of undergoing hand or wrist arthroplasty or arthrodesis and 90% higher odds of having tendon reconstructive pro-cedures.[11] This is in contrast to another population at risk for RA outcome inequities, Indigenous populations, who continue to experience colonized health systems, racism, and stereotyping, resulting in decreased surgical access for conditions including secondary osteoarthritis.[12]

DISPARITIES IN ACCESS TO MEDICATIONS

Several populations, including those determined by socioeconomic status, race or ethnicity, age, gender, and geographic location of residence, have been identified to have variations in medication access. Older studies have reported on access to disease-modifying antirheumatic drugs (DMARDs). In a cohort comparison study of patients with access to a rheumatology clinic in a public county hospital providing care primarily to minority, disadvantaged or uninsured patients with RA, relative to those receiving rheumatology care at a private clinic, yet with both sites affiliated with the same medical school, a difference of 4.5 years for DMARD initiation between private and public clinic attendees, and 6 years based on White and non-White ethnicity, was estimated.[13] Health care Effectiveness Data and Information Set data from the National Committee for Quality Assurance confirmed decreased DMARD receipt for several populations at risk for inequities, including for those older than 65 years, men, Black ethnicity, those residing in particular geographic areas of the United States, along with low personal income, residing in socioeconomically disadvantaged neighborhoods, and enrollment in for-profit plans.[14] In an American cohort, albeit with self-reported RA, Medicaid patients aged 18 to 64 years had significantly increased odds of receiving NSAIDs, however with only a 26% odds of receiving nonbiological DMARDs.[10]

The issue of biological therapy availability to population groups with low socioeconomic status is an even more acute concern given the cost of these therapies to payers. Using Truven's MarketScan Commercial Claims and Encounters and Medicare Supplemental and Coordination of Benefits data, increasing age; residence in the American Midwest, Northeast, and West regions; and having Medical supplemental insurance were associated with reduced odds of tumor necrosis factor (TNF)-alpha inhibitor treatment initiation in patients on nonbiological monotherapy, whereas age alone was a negative predictor of initiation if on combination nonbiologic therapy.[15] In the aforementioned American cohort with self-reported RA, Medicaid patients aged 18 to 64 years had just 9% the odds of receiving biological therapy compared with patients with private insurance.[10] In the first 10 years of biological therapy availability in Canada, only 10% of patients exposed to DMARD therapy with cost coverage through the Non-Insured Health Benefits branch of Health Canada, representing those who have retained First Nations Status through the Indian Act, went on to receive a biological therapy,[16] whereas at that point in time approximately 24% of the general population with RA in Ontario were being treated with these strategies.[17]

Receiving biological therapy is not only influenced by socioeconomic status; in a study comparing the prevalence of biological therapy use between patients in a single-payer health system (Veterans Affairs Rheumatoid Arthritis Registry) and those with a mix of self-paid insurance, Medicare, and Medicaid, biological therapy use was highest in White patients with insurance coverage, even compared with White patients in the single-payer health system, and for patients who were of non-White ethnicity, for similar levels of RA disease activity.[18] In contrast, rural residence may afford increased access, with a nearly 2-fold increased probability of initiation of biological therapy once individual and contextual factors were considered in an American population.[19]

Therapeutic persistence was not found to vary by rural residence in a Canadian cohort, either for DMARD therapy or biological therapy.[20] However, rural location of care has been found to inform the selection of route of administration of medication. In a Canadian study, receiving rheumatology care in a rural area was associated with a nearly 4-fold increase in initiating a TNF-alpha inhibitor biologic over a non-TNF-alpha strategy, with also nearly uniquely being started on subcutaneous rather than intravenous therapy, with adjustment for gender, age, smoking, disease duration, function, concurrent use of antiinflammatories, academic affiliated site, time period, and number of comorbidities.[21] The impact of these trends on disease activity and outcomes is not known but raises concerns for prescribing bias favoring convenience for rural patients.

PATIENT EXPERIENCE AND PERFORMANCE IN QUALITY-OF-CARE INDICATORS

Relatively little information on the experience of rheumatology care for persons from populations at risk for inequities in RA care is available. A study from Saskatchewan, Canada used qualitative research methodology to explore rural patients' experiences of RA care. Although access to care was the greatest concern raised, patients with longer travel times had higher satisfaction with their health care appointments, suggesting that strong patient-provider relationships are important for a good-quality care experience.[22]

One approach in examining care accessibility is through evaluation of Ambulatory Care Sensitive Conditions (ACSC), which is applied as a metric reflecting that appropriate access to quality healthcare services will prevent costly hospitalizations for exacerbations of chronic diseases.[23] ACSCs are not defined in rheumatology, and as hospitalization for RA is no longer a frequent outcome, contact with the urgent or emergent health care system may be used as an indicator of poor specialty access and appropriate care. This is supported by research that documented that after attempts at self-management, patients with RA will seek primary care assessment or attend the emergency department if their rheumatologist is unable to accommodate them in a timely fashion.[24] Inequity concerns are suggested to also be reflected in emergency department use. In the state of Nebraska from 2007 to 2012, emergency department visits for arthritis and other related conditions provided information that female gender and older age were associated with higher visit rates.[25]

Exploration of established indicators of quality of care, such as adherence to system-level performance measures in populations at risk for inequities in outcomes, and patient satisfaction with rheumatology care experiences, should be embedded within further research and quality improvement studies. Room should also be made to define indicators more relevant to the populations served. An example of this comes from an activity the Public Health Agency of Canada undertook, called the "Canadian Best Practices Initiative,", to compile promising health promotion and chronic disease interventions throughout the nation. It was realized that the framework by which the agency sought to identify exemplary programs did not align well with Indigenous community knowledge and approaches. This led to assembling expertise and the creation of a measurement framework that incorporated Indigenous values on interventions.[26]

MODELS OF CARE AND TREATMENT APPROACHES TO SUPPORT BETTER RHEUMATOID ARTHRITIS OUTCOMES FOR POPULATIONS AT RISK OF INEQUITIES

Quality improvement approaches that engage those required to make sustainable meaningful changes have been described as successful in populations facing RA outcome inequities. In California, a pay-for-performance initiative instigated an interprofessional approach in a clinic serving urban racially/ethnically and socioeconomically diverse patients with RA.[27] Foci for redesigned clinical processes included vaccination completion, disease activity monitoring, latent tuberculosis infection screening before biological use and reproductive health counseling. Enhancing workflow, engaging nonphysician providers, and managing practice variation were instrumental in achieving targets. In Australia, Mitchell and colleagues[28] described a modified continuous quality improvement approach to improve culturally and socially inclusive care within rural health services, requiring deep engagement of health system staff to reflect on dominant discourses, understanding the need for and engaging in change, including community members and shifting organizational culture to support delivery of culturally inclusive health care.

Models of care that facilitate access and continuity of care are critical to develop and implement. Described models include distributed models of care, including provision of rheumatology care in locales more convenient and accessible to patients,[29] and using technology such as telehealth to connect with persons in remote locations.[30] System capacity may be enhanced by using allied health professionals, including Advanced Clinician Practitioner in Arthritis Care (ACPAC)-trained practitioners[31] and supporting nurse-led care,[32] which have been offered as solutions to meet increased patient volumes due to increasing the number of initial assessments for early diagnosis and frequent reassessments. Lessons may also be learned from other areas of medicine. Innovative cross-sector studies providing social service need screening, patient navigation, and housing supports are under evaluation for feasibility and ability to improve health outcomes.[33]

The care provision in clinics must also ensure culturally safe environments, either through enhanced knowledge and skills in communication strategies with defined patient groups,[34] using trauma-informed care strategies,[35] or increasing the number of rheumatologists from the populations at risk for inequity,[36] as this is likely to increase relationship building and understanding.

Treatment decision support is another important consideration. Health literacy and power differentials affect medication adherence. The preferred approach to steer away from paternalistic medicine is shared decision-making, which encompasses tools and approaches to increase patient engagement in decision-making, through identification of benefits, negatives, and patient preferences for clinical decisions and has been shown to result in better health outcomes.[37] In a study that enrolled patients with RA exposed to therapy, a low-literacy medication guide and decision aid was beneficial to improve knowledge and reduce decisional conflict for those of older age, who were immigrants, who were non-English speakers, had less than high school education, had limited health literacy, and were from a racial minority group.[38]

SUMMARY

This article introduces the literature base on disparities in RA care for populations at risk of inequities and suggestions for mechanisms by which the rheumatology community could support these populations. These activities call on our need to drive advocacy, redistribute privilege, and launch collaborative initiatives within systems and clinics to close care gaps, and consider which activities we prioritize for ensuring all patients can secure optimal RA outcomes.

ACKNOWLEDGEMENTS

Dr. Barnabe is a Canada Research Chair in Rheumatoid Arthritis and Autoimmune Diseases, Canadian Institutes of Health Research.

REFERENCES

1. Chatzidionysiou K, Sfikakis PP. Low rates of remission with methotrexate monotherapy in rheumatoid arthritis: review of randomised controlled trials could point towards a paradigm shift. RMD Open 2019;5(2):e000993.

2. Smolen JS, Landewé RBM, Bijlsma JWJ, et al. EULAR recommendations for the management of rheumatoid arthritis with synthetic and biological disease-modifying antirheumatic drugs: 2019 update. Ann Rheum Dis 2020;79(6):685–99.

3. Singh JA, Saag KG, Bridges SL Jr, et al. 2015 American College of Rheumatology guideline for the treatment of rheumatoid arthritis. Arthritis Rheumatol 2016; 68(1):1–26.

4. Barber CE, Marshall DA, Mosher DP, et al. Development of system-level performance measures for evaluation of models of care for inflammatory arthritis in Canada. J Rheumatol 2016;43(3):530–40.

5. Lorenc T, Oliver K. Adverse effects of public health interventions: a conceptual framework. J Epidemiol Community Health 2014;68(3):288–90.

6. Petkovic J, Epstein J, Buchbinder R, et al. Toward ensuring health equity: readability and cultural equivalence of OMERACT patient-reported outcome measures. J Rheumatol 2015;42(12):2448–59.

7. Petkovic J, Barton JL, Flurey C, et al. Health equity considerations for developing and reporting patient-reported outcomes in clinical trials: a report from the OMERACT Equity Special Interest Group. J Rheumatol 2017;44(11):1727–33.

8. Widdifield J, Paterson JM, Bernatsky S, et al. Access to rheumatologists among patients with newly diagnosed rheumatoid arthritis in a Canadian universal public healthcare system. BMJ Open 2014;4(1):e003888.

9. Polinski JM, Brookhart MA, Ayanian JZ, et al. Relationships between driving distance, rheumatoid arthritis diagnosis, and disease-modifying antirheumatic drug receipt. Arthritis Care Res (Hoboken) 2014;66(11):1634–43.

10. Cifaldi M, Renaud J, Ganguli A, et al. Disparities in care by insurance status for individuals with rheumatoid arthritis: analysis of the medical expenditure panel survey, 2006-2009. Curr Med Res Opin 2016;32(12):2029–37.

11. Zhong L, Chung KC, Baser O, et al. Variation in rheumatoid hand and wrist surgery among medicare beneficiaries: a population-based cohort study. J Rheumatol 2015;42(3):429–36.

12. Loyola-Sanchez A, Hurd K, Barnabe C. Healthcare utilization for arthritis by indigenous populations of Australia, Canada, New Zealand, and the United States: A systematic review. Semin Arthritis Rheum 2017;46(5):665–74.

13. Suarez-Almazor ME, Berrios-Rivera JP, Cox V, et al. Initiation of disease-modifying antirheumatic drug therapy in minority and disadvantaged patients with rheumatoid arthritis. J Rheumatol 2007;34(12):2400–7.

14. Schmajuk G, Trivedi AN, Solomon DH, et al. Receipt of disease-modifying antirheumatic drugs among patients with rheumatoid arthritis in Medicare managed care plans. JAMA 2011;305(5):480–6.

15. Desai RJ, Rao JK, Hansen RA, et al. Predictors of treatment initiation with tumor necrosis factor-α inhibitors in patients with rheumatoid arthritis. J Manag Care Spec Pharm 2014;20(11):1110–20.

16. Barnabe C, Healy B, Portolesi A, et al. Claims for disease-modifying therapy by Alberta non-insured health benefits clients. BMC Health Serv Res 2016;16:1–8.

17. Widdifield J, Bernatsky S, Paterson JM, et al. Accuracy of Canadian health administrative databases in identifying patients with rheumatoid arthritis: a validation study using the medical records of rheumatologists. Arthritis Care Res (Hoboken) 2013;65(10):1582–91.

18. Kerr GS, Swearingen C, Mikuls TR, et al. Use of biologic therapy in racial minorities with rheumatoid arthritis from 2 US Health Care Systems. J Clin Rheumatol 2017;23(1):12–8.

19. Yelin E, Tonner C, Kim SC, et al. Sociodemographic, disease, health system, and contextual factors affecting the initiation of biologic agents in rheumatoid arthritis: a longitudinal study. Arthritis Care Res (Hoboken) 2014;66(7):980–9.

20. Ahluwalia V, Rampakakis E, Movahedi M, et al. Predictors of patient decision to discontinue anti-rheumatic medication in patients with rheumatoid arthritis: results from the Ontario best practices research initiative. Clin Rheumatol 2017; 36(11):2421–30.

21. Movahedi M, Joshi R, Rampakakis E, et al. Impact of residential area on the management of rheumatoid arthritis patients initiating their first biologic DMARD: Results from the Ontario Best Practices Research Initiative (OBRI). Medicine (Baltimore) 2019;98(20):e15517.

22. Nair BV, Schuler R, Stewart S, et al. Self-reported barriers to healthcare access for rheumatoid arthritis patients in rural and northern saskatchewan: a mixed methods study. Musculoskeletal Care 2016;14(4):243–51.

23. Vuik SI, Fontana G, Mayer E, et al. Do hospitalisations for ambulatory care sensitive conditions reflect low access to primary care? An observational cohort study of primary care usage prior to hospitalisation. BMJ Open 2017;7(8): e015704.

24. Flurey CA, Morris M, Pollock J, et al. A Q-methodology study of flare help-seeking behaviours and different experiences of daily life in rheumatoid arthritis. BMC Musculoskelet Disord 2014;15:364.

25. Han GM, Michaud K, Yu F, et al. Increasing public health burden of arthritis and other rheumatic conditions and comorbidity: results from a statewide health surveillance system, 2007-2012. Arthritis Care Res (Hoboken) 2016;68(10): 1417–27.

26. Public Health Agency of Canada. Ways Tried and True. Aboriginal Methodological Framework for the Canadian Best Practices Initiative. Ottawa (Ontario): Government of Canada, Public Health Agency of Canada: 2015.

27. Aguirre A, Trupin L, Margaretten M, et al. Using process improvement and systems redesign to improve rheumatology care quality in a safety net clinic. J Rheumatol 2020. https://doi.org/10.3899/jrheum.190472.

28. Mitchell O, Malatzky C, Bourke L, et al. A modified Continuous Quality Improvement approach to improve culturally and socially inclusive care within rural health services. Aust J Rural Health 2018;26(3):206–10.

29. Nagaraj S, Kargard M, Hemmelgarn B, et al. Effectiveness of an outreach model of care for rheumatology specialty clinics to an on-reserve first nations community. Int J Indig Health 2018;13(1):156–66.

30. McDougall JA, Ferucci ED, Glover J, et al. Telerheumatology: a systematic review. Arthritis Care Res (Hoboken) 2017;69(10):1546–57.

31. Passalent LA, Kennedy C, Warmington K, et al. System integration and clinical utilization of the Advanced Clinician Practitioner in Arthritis Care (ACPAC) Program-Trained Extended Role Practitioners in Ontario: a two-year, system-level evaluation. Healthc Policy 2013;8(4):56–70.

32. Garner S, Lopatina E, Rankin JA, et al. Nurse-led care for patients with rheumatoid arthritis: a systematic review of the effect on quality of care. J Rheumatol 2017;44(6):757–65.

33. Fichtenberg CM, Alley DE, Mistry KB. Improving social needs intervention research: key questions for advancing the field. Am J Prev Med 2019;57(6S1): S47–54.

34. Thurston WE, Coupal S, Jones CA, et al. Discordant indigenous and provider frames explain challenges in improving access to arthritis care: a

qualitative study using constructivist grounded theory. Int J Equity Health 2014;13(1):46.

35. Roberts SJ, Chandler GE, Kalmakis K. A model for trauma-informed primary care. J Am Assoc Nurse Pract 2019;31(2):139–44.

36. Truth and Reconciliation Commission of Canada. Truth and Reconciliation Commission of Canada: Calls to Action. Winnipeg (Manitoba): Truth and Reconciliation Commission of Canada: 2015.

37. Stacey D, Hill S, McCaffery K, et al. Shared Decision Making Interventions: Theoretical and Empirical Evidence with Implications for Health Literacy. Stud Health Technol Inform 2017;240:263–83.

38. Barton JL, Trupin L, Schillinger D, et al. Use of low-literacy decision aid to enhance knowledge and reduce decisional conflict among a diverse population of adults with rheumatoid arthritis: results of a pilot study. Arthritis Care Res (Hoboken) 2016;68(7):889–98.

Gender and Ethnic Inequities in Gout Burden and Management

Andrea Garcia Guillén, MD[a,1],
Leanne Te Karu, DipPharm, MHSc(Hons)[b,c],
Jasvinder A. Singh, MD, MPH[d,e,f], Nicola Dalbeth, MD, FRACP[g,h],*

KEYWORDS

- Gout • Urate • Equity • Disparities • Gender • Ethnicity

KEY POINTS

- Women, African-Americans in the United States, Māori (Indigenous New Zealanders), and Pacific people living in Aotearoa/New Zealand experience inequitable gout care.
- Barriers to effective gout management occur at several levels, including health care practitioners, health organizations, and the health system.
- A focus on culturally safe health care that builds health literacy and removes barriers to continuous urate-lowering therapy is needed to eliminate inequity for people with gout.

INTRODUCTION

Gout is a chronic disease of monosodium urate crystal deposition that typically presents as intermittent flares of severe inflammatory arthritis.[1] Poorly controlled gout has an important impact on musculoskeletal function, health-related quality of life (HRQOL),[2] and productivity.[3] Gout is also associated with comorbid conditions

Funding Statement: A.G. Guillén is supported by the Spanish Foundation for Rheumatology and the Catalan Society of Rheumatology.
[a] Department of Medicine, University of Auckland, Auckland, New Zealand; [b] Ngā Kaitiaki o te Puna Rongoā o Aotearoa, Taupō, New Zealand; [c] School of Pharmacy, University of Otago, PO Box 56, Dunedin 9054, New Zealand; [d] Medicine Service, VA Medical Center; [e] Department of Medicine at the School of Medicine, University of Alabama at Birmingham, Birmingham, AL, USA; [f] Department of Epidemiology at the School of Public Health, University of Alabama at Birmingham, Faculty Office Tower 805B, 510 20th Street South, Birmingham, AL 35294, USA; [g] Department of Medicine, Faculty of Medical and Health Sciences, University of Auckland, 85 Park Road, Grafton, Auckland 1023, New Zealand; [h] Department of Rheumatology, Auckland District Health Board, Auckland, New Zealand
[1] Present address: Hospital de la Santa Creu i Sant Pau, Sant Antoni Maria Claret, 167, Barcelona 08025, Spain.
* Corresponding author. Department of Medicine, Faculty of Medical and Health Sciences, University of Auckland, 85 Park Road, Grafton, Auckland 1023, New Zealand.
E-mail address: n.dalbeth@auckland.ac.nz

including cardiovascular disease, chronic kidney disease, and diabetes, and a premature mortality gap.[4,5]

The central strategy for effective gout management is continuous urate-lowering therapy to achieve monosodium urate crystal dissolution, suppression of gout flares, and prevention of joint damage.[6] Although effective and low-cost urate-lowering therapy, such as allopurinol, has been available since the 1960s,[7] disparities in gout management exist. In this review, we summarize the evidence for gender and racial disparities in gout management, identify factors that may contribute to these disparities, and describe potential strategies to eliminate inequity in gout outcomes.

GENDER DISPARITIES

Gout is less common in women than in men. Recent estimates of gout prevalence for women living in the United States were 2.7%, compared with 5.2% of men,[8] and in Taiwan, gout affected 3.2% of women and 9.3% of men.[9] Compared with men, women with gout are generally older, have greater burden of comorbidities, and use more diuretics.[10] Women with gout have an excellent response to the urate-lowering therapies including allopurinol and febuxostat.[11]

Differences in the quality of care according to gender have been reported (**Table 1**). Women are less likely to receive allopurinol,[8,10,12] and more likely to receive glucocorticoids and nonsteroidal anti-inflammatory drugs (NSAIDs).[10] The reasons for different prescribing patterns between men and women has not been examined in detail. In general, long-term urate-lowering therapy is recommended for patients with frequent gout flares or tophi, and it is possible that some women with gout do not require or choose not to take long-term urate-lowering therapy because of infrequent flares or mild disease. However, women with gout report similar frequency of flares and greater

Table 1
Studies reporting quality of gout care for women

Study	Population	Outcome	Results
Harrold et al,[10] 2006	6133 patients in US health maintenance organizations	Receiving allopurinol	Women vs men: odds ratio, 0.78; 95% CI, 0.67–0.90
		Receiving glucocorticoids	Women vs men: odds ratio, 1.30; 95% CI, 1.12–1.50
		Receiving nonsteroidal anti-inflammatory drugs	Women vs men: odds ratio, 1.68; 95% CI, 1.29–2.18
		Serum urate monitoring within 6 mo after starting urate-lowering therapy	Women vs men: odds ratio, 1.36; 95% CI, 1.11–1.67
Harrold et al,[12] 2017	1273 US national cohort of gout patients cared for by rheumatologists	Receiving any urate-lowering therapy	77% women, 83% men
		Receiving allopurinol	51% women, 64% men
		Receiving febuxostat	26% women, 17% men
Chen-Xu et al,[8] 2019	5467 participants in the NHANES 2015–2016	Current urate-lowering therapy use	15.5% women, 43.0% men

Abbreviations: CI, confidence interval; NHANES, National Health and Nutrition Examination Survey.

activity limitation compared with men with gout, even after adjusting for comorbidities and duration of gout,[4] suggesting that less severe disease does not fully explain the observed prescribing differences between genders.

Qualitative research has shown that gout has a major impact on quality of life for men and women.[13] Women with gout are concerned about dependency, joint deformity, and difficulty with footwear.[13] Women with gout also describe difficulty finding relevant information for them, because information is targeted to men.[14] The diagnostic process can be uncertain and may be delayed because of lack of awareness of gout in women by health providers.[14] Gout has a major impact on women's identity and on their roles and relationships.[14] Perceptions about gout as a "man's disease" may contribute to stigmatization and embarrassment in women with gout, which can create barriers to seeking medical care for gout.[15]

RACIAL/ETHNIC DISPARITIES: UNITED STATES

In the United States, contemporary prevalence estimates of gout are 4.8% in non-Hispanic African-Americans, 4.0% in non-Hispanic Whites, and 2.0% in Hispanics.[8] African-Americans with gout have greater impact of gout and a lower HRQOL compared with White patients with gout.[16] In clinical trial settings, African-Americans with gout have similar urate-lowering responses to allopurinol and febuxostat compared with White patients with gout.[17]

Despite the higher impact of disease and documented efficacy of urate-lowering treatment, studies over the last two decades have shown that African-Americans with gout are less likely to be prescribed allopurinol and are more likely to have interruptions in allopurinol prescribing compared with White Americans with gout (**Table 2**).[8,18,19] Most recent estimates show that urate-lowering therapy is prescribed in 26.5% non-Hispanic Black adults, 35.0% in non-Hispanic White adults, and 57.7% in Hispanic adults in the United States.[8] Compared with White Americans on allopurinol, African-American veterans on allopurinol had significantly lower adjusted odds of achieving target serum urate.[20]

In qualitative studies, African-Americans with gout reported severe pain during gout flares and significantly associated emotional burden and dietary restriction

| Table 2 |||||
| Studies reporting quality of gout care for African-Americans in the United States |||||
Study	Population	Outcome	Results
Krishnan et al,[18] 2008	3.9 million ambulatory care visits	Allopurinol prescription	African-American vs White: odds ratio, 0.18; 95% CI, 0.04–0.78
Solomon et al,[19] 2008	9823 older adults enrolled in a pharmacy benefit program	Inconsistent prescribing of urate-lowering therapy	African-American vs White: odds ratio, 1.86; 95% CI, 1.52–2.27
Singh et al,[20] 2019	41,153 patients on allopurinol in the Veterans Affairs health care system	Achieving target serum urate (<6 mg/dL)	African-American vs White: odds ratio, 0.84 (0.80–0.88)
Chen-Xu et al,[8] 2019	5467 participants in the NHANES 2015–2016	Urate-lowering therapy prescription	26.5% non-Hispanic Black adults, 35.0% non-Hispanic White adults, 57.7% Hispanic adults

caused by gout.[13] Doubts about the effectiveness of urate-lowering therapy, concerns about the cost and side effects of therapy, impact of concomitant medications, and pill size were noted to be barriers to medication adherence.[21] African-Americans reporting low adherence to urate-lowering therapy describe the lack of communication from physicians about the usefulness of therapy, whereas patients with high adherence report greater understanding of the disease and its treatment.[21]

ETHNIC DISPARITIES: AOTEAROA/NEW ZEALAND

It has been documented for decades that hyperuricemia and gout is common throughout Polynesia.[22,23] In contemporary Aotearoa/New Zealand, gout is estimated to affect 8.5% Māori (Indigenous New Zealanders), 13.9% Pacific peoples (eg, Tongan, Sāmoan, Cook Island Māori, Niuean), and 4.2% other New Zealanders (eg, New Zealand European, Asian, Indian).[24] Compared with other New Zealanders with gout, Māori and Pacific peoples have earlier age of onset, higher flare frequency, and more features of joint inflammation.[25] This may be caused by population-specific genetic variants contributing to hyperuricemia and gout[26,27]; higher prevalence of comorbid conditions that contribute to hyperuricemia, such as kidney disease; or undertreatment with urate-lowering therapy throughout the disease course. Early in the course of disease, Māori and Pacific peoples experience greater pain and activity limitation and lower HRQOL.[25] Māori and Pacific peoples are also disproportionately prescribed NSAIDs for gout management and have high rates of hospital admission for management of severe gout.[24,28,29]

Despite the high prevalence and severity of disease in Māori and in Pacific peoples living in Aotearoa/New Zealand, these groups are less likely to receive effective preventive therapy in the form of continuous urate-lowering therapy than other New Zealanders (**Table 3**).[24,28] In 2016, continuous urate-lowering therapy for three-quarters or four-quarters in a year was dispensed to 34.9% Pacific peoples, 40.4% Māori, and 44.4% other New Zealanders with gout.[24]

Qualitative studies have also demonstrated the severe impact of gout in Aotearoa/New Zealand. Māori and Pacific men with gout describe extreme pain, dependency on whānau (family) members during flares, isolation, and work disability.[30] For Māori, gout has a huge, negative impact, causing overwhelming suffering.[31] The burden of disease of gout can ripple through to whānau, having negative consequences on relationships and employment. Māori with gout experience receiving little information about the cause or appropriate management of gout from health care practitioners.[31]

The experience of gout for Māori, the Indigenous people of Aotearoa/New Zealand, has particular importance. Under Article 3 of Te Tiriti o Waitangi (The Treaty of Waitangi[a]), the founding document of Aotearoa/New Zealand, Māori are guaranteed the same rights and privileges as non-Māori, which includes "at least the same level of health as non-Māori."[32] In addition, Aotearoa/New Zealand became a signatory to the United Nations Declaration on the Rights of Indigenous Peoples in 2010; under Article 24 of the United Nations Declaration, Māori, as the Indigenous people of Aotearoa/New Zealand, "have an equal right to the enjoyment of the highest attainable standard of physical and mental health." The inequity in gout care for Māori, who are disproportionately affected by this disease, indicates failing of obligations under Te Tiriti o Waitangi and the United Nations Declaration.[24]

---

[a] This is a translation of the title of the document. There are important differences in meaning between the Māori language and English language texts.

Table 3
Studies reporting quality of gout care for Māori and Pacific Peoples in Aotearoa/New Zealand

Study	Population	Outcome	Results
Jackson et al,[29] 2014	114,703 New Zealanders with gout (national administrative data 2011)	Dispensed any urate-lowering therapy	67% Māori, 63% Pacific peoples, 71% other New Zealanders
		Hospital admissions for gout	1.7% Māori, 1.6% Pacific peoples, 0.6% other New Zealanders
		Laboratory testing for serum urate in the 6 mo following dispensing	33% Māori, 37% Pacific peoples, 34% other New Zealanders
Dalbeth et al,[28] 2016	164,169 New Zealanders with gout (national administrative data 2014)	Regularly dispensed urate-lowering therapy	39% Māori, 33% Pacific peoples, 43% other New Zealanders
Dalbeth et al,[24] 2018	182,013 New Zealanders with gout (national administrative data 2016)	Dispensed nonsteroidal anti-inflammatory drugs	40.8% Māori, 46.7% Pacific peoples, 33.9% other New Zealanders
		Regularly dispensed urate-lowering therapy	40.3% Māori, 34.9% Pacific peoples, 44.3% other New Zealanders
		Hospital admissions because of gout (rate per 100.000 population)	114.5 Māori, 202.2 Pacific peoples, 24.5 other New Zealanders

WHAT IS DRIVING INEQUITY IN GOUT MANAGEMENT?

Many of the factors that contribute to health inequity, including social determinants of health, institutional racism, sexism, and the pervasive negative impact of colonization, likely contribute to the disparities in gout management described previously. For example, financial barriers to and through the health care system may contribute to the observed ethnic disparities in gout management in Aotearoa/New Zealand. Data from a recent Primary Care Patient Experience Survey in Aotearoa/New Zealand showed that 29% Māori participants and 29% Pacific peoples participants did not visit a general practitioner or nurse because of cost, compared with 19% New Zealand European participants.[24] Furthermore, 24% of Māori participants and 22% of Pacific participants identified cost as a barrier to pick up prescriptions, compared with 7% New Zealand European participants.[24] In addition, there are specific challenges to gout management that may contribute to poor quality of care.

In western cultures, historical depictions of gout over many centuries have focused on gout as a self-inflicted and humorous disease of lifestyle excess.[33] These beliefs about gout are commonly held by health care professionals and the wider community,[31,33,34] despite contemporary scientific understanding about the biologic causes for gout (including aging, chronic kidney disease, medications, and genetic contributors). Prevailing beliefs about the cause of gout can contribute to stigmatization and embarrassment that is experienced by people with gout,[35] particularly women with gout,[14] and Māori and Pacific peoples.[30,35] In a qualitative study of Māori with gout, all participants believed or had been informed that gout is caused by dietary factors, leading to feelings of self-blame and blame from partners and employers.[31] For people with gout, stigmatization negatively interferes with seeking health care and treatment adherence.[35] Historical western views about gout as a disease that is primarily caused by diet can also contribute to excessive focus on unproven strategies for gout,[36] rather than effective long-term medications.

The presentation of gout as an acute flaring condition with asymptomatic intercritical periods can also reinforce the belief of health care professionals, patients, and families that gout is an acute illness that is present only during the flare, rather than a chronic disease of urate crystal deposition that requires long-term continuous urate-lowering therapy.[34] Qualitative studies of Māori and Pacific men with gout highlight the importance of ongoing relationships with health care professionals who can effectively communicate about the underlying basis of gout, providing the rationale for continuous urate-lowering therapy.[30,31] The requirements of health care systems to access medical appointments, laboratory tests, and pharmacy care exert substantial health literacy demands and contribute to a fragmented and burdensome patient experience.[37]

Recruitment approaches in clinical trials of new therapeutic agents for gout may further exacerbate inequities in gout management. In large phase 3 clinical trials that have contributed to Food and Drug Administration approvals of medications for gout in the last 20 years, most study participants have been white men (**Table 4**). The underrepresentation of women and non-White trial participants limits the understanding of treatment responses (efficacy and safety) in these groups.

STRATEGIES TO ACHIEVE HEALTH EQUITY IN GOUT

Strategies to improve the quality of gout care have been described within primary care, the setting in which most gout is managed. These approaches have included practice management improvement interventions[38–40] and packages of care led by nurses and pharmacists.[41–45] The most successful strategies take a health literacy approach, exploring the individual patient's beliefs about gout, supporting understanding that gout is a chronic disease of crystal deposition, and focusing on behavior change to take continuous urate-lowering therapy.[37] Health literacy approaches that reduce barriers to chronic care management, with point-of-care serum urate testing,

Table 4
Characteristics of participants in phase 3 clinical trials contributing to regulatory approvals for gout in the United States since 2009

Study, Year	Total Participants (n)	Male, n (%)	White, n (%)
Becker et al,[51] 2005	762	729 (95.6)	587 (77.0)
Schumacher Jr et al,[52] 2008	1072	1002 (93.5)	835 (77.9)
Becker et al,[53] 2010	2269	2141 (94.4)	1863 (82.1)
Terkeltaub et al,[54] 2010	185	176 (95.1)	153 (82.7)
Sundy et al,[55] 2011	225	173 (81.6)	143 (67.5)
Saag et al,[56] 2017	603	567 (94.0)	460 (76.3)
Bardin et al,[57] 2017	610	587 (96.2)	482 (79.0)
Dalbeth et al,[58] 2017	324	309 (95.4)	259 (79.9)
Tausche et al,[59] 2017	214	195 (91.1)	175 (81.8)

prescription reminders, and regular follow-up, can lead to major improvements in persistence with urate-lowering therapy, improved serum urate lowering, fewer gout flares, and improved HRQOL.

Although these programs have been reported for the general population, most studies examining gout quality improvement interventions have underrepresentation of women and non-White participants. For women, existing educational resources are not tailored to their needs.[14] Furthermore, preferences in how information about gout is communicated may vary in different ethnic groups. For example, Māori prefer information about gout to be kanohi-ki-te-kanohi (face-to-face) in the presence of whānau.[46] Māori also report having lower preference for communicating about gout from a general practitioner/specialist and in written form.[47] Differences in health care delivery needs and preferences are important when developing culturally safe strategies that focus on health equity for people with gout.

One example of a successful project is the Gout Stop program, an interprovider collaborative project developed for primary care in Northland, Aotearoa/New Zealand.[48] This program includes a prescription pack protocol for starting urate-lowering therapy, serum urate point-of-care testing by community pharmacists, gout educators, and an Indigenous community support worker (Kaiāwhina) who provides education and support to patients and whānau. A target of greater than 70% Māori and Pacific patient participation in the program was prespecified to address the goal of reducing health inequities. From 2015 to 2017, 887 patients enrolled in the program, of whom 67% were Māori and 4% were Pacific peoples. Following program completion, 68% of Māori and Pacific patients and 65% of non-Māori/non-Pacific patients continued to take allopurinol. Moreover, data from the Health Quality & Safety Commission New Zealand Atlas of Healthcare Variation showed than within 1 year of commencing the program, allopurinol use in Northland was higher and NSAIDs use lower than the national average, particularly for Māori patients.[48] This program highpoints the potential benefits of a culturally safe, multidisciplinary team approach centered within primary care to facilitate equitable gout outcomes.

SUMMARY

Although individual health practitioner and organization-led approaches play an important role in eliminating health inequity for people with gout, broader contributors to inequitable outcomes for people with gout should be recognized. Integrated action across sectors is required to address the unfair distribution of the social determinants of health.[49] Health systems should focus on equity as an integral component of quality,[32] including building and maintaining a workforce that is culturally safe.[50] Prioritizing equity throughout the health system is likely to lead to major improvements in outcome for people with gout.

DISCLOSURE

A.G. Guillén and L. Te Karu have no disclosures. J.A. Singh has received consultant fees from Crealta/Horizon, MediSYS, Fidia, UBM LLC, Trio health, Medscape, WebMD, Clinical Care options, Clearview health care partners, Putnam associates, Focus forward, Navigant consulting, Spherix, Practice Point communications, the National Institutes of Health, and the American College of Rheumatology (ACR). J.A. Singh owns stock options in Amarin pharmaceuticals and Viking therapeutics. J.A. Singh is on the speaker's bureau of Simply Speaking. J.A. Singh is a member of the executive of OMERACT, an organization that develops outcome measures in rheumatology and receives arms-length funding from 12 companies. J.A. Singh serves on the Food and Drug Administration Arthritis Advisory Committee. J.A. Singh is the chair of the Veterans Affairs Rheumatology Field Advisory Committee. J.A. Singh is the editor and the Director of the UAB Cochrane Musculoskeletal Group Satellite Center on Network Meta-analysis. J.A. Singh previously served as a member of the following committees: member, the ACR Annual Meeting Planning Committee and Quality of Care Committees; the Chair of the ACR Meet-the-Professor, Workshop, and Study Group Subcommittee; and the cochair of the ACR Criteria and Response Criteria subcommittee. N. Dalbeth has received fees from Janssen, AbbVie, CymaBay, AstraZeneca, Crealta, Takeda, Kowa, Horizon, Hengrui, Dyve Biosciences, Arthrosi, Selecta, bpac, the Health Research Council of New Zealand, UpToDate, Oxford University Press, the Pharmaceutical Society of New Zealand, the Spanish Society for Rheumatology, the Asia Pacific Gout Consortium, and the ACR. Her institution has received research grants from the Health Research Council of New Zealand, the Auckland Medical Research Foundation, PHARMAC, AstraZeneca, and Amgen.

REFERENCES

1. Faires JS, McCarty DJ. Acute arthritis in man and dog after intrasynovial injection of sodium urate crystals. Lancet 1962;280:682–5.
2. Singh JA, Strand V. Gout is associated with more comorbidities, poorer health-related quality of life and higher healthcare utilisation in US veterans. Ann Rheum Dis 2008;67(9):1310–6.
3. Kleinman NL, Brook RA, Patel PA, et al. The impact of gout on work absence and productivity. Value Health 2007;10(4):231–7.
4. Richette P, Clerson P, Perissin L, et al. Revisiting comorbidities in gout: a cluster analysis. Ann Rheum Dis 2015;74(1):142–7.
5. Fisher MC, Rai SK, Lu N, et al. The unclosing premature mortality gap in gout: a general population-based study. Ann Rheum Dis 2017;76(7):1289–94.
6. Richette P, Doherty M, Pascual E, et al. 2016 updated EULAR evidence-based recommendations for the management of gout. Ann Rheum Dis 2017;76(1): 29–42.
7. Yue TF, Gutman AB. Effect of allopurinol (4-hydroxypyrazolo-(3,4-d)pyrimidine) on serum and urinary uric acid in primary and secondary gout. Am J Med 1964;37:885–98.
8. Chen-Xu M, Yokose C, Rai SK, et al. Contemporary prevalence of gout and hyperuricemia in the united states and decadal trends: the National Health and Nutrition Examination Survey, 2007-2016. Arthritis Rheumatol 2019;71(6):991–9.
9. Kuo CF, Grainge MJ, See LC, et al. Epidemiology and management of gout in Taiwan: a nationwide population study. Arthritis Res Ther 2015;17:13.
10. Harrold LR, Yood RA, Mikuls TR, et al. Sex differences in gout epidemiology: evaluation and treatment. Ann Rheum Dis 2006;65(10):1368–72.
11. Chohan S, Becker MA, MacDonald PA, et al. Women with gout: efficacy and safety of urate-lowering with febuxostat and allopurinol. Arthritis Care Res (Hoboken) 2012;64(2):256–61.
12. Harrold LR, Etzel CJ, Gibofsky A, et al. Sex differences in gout characteristics: tailoring care for women and men. BMC Musculoskelet Disord 2017;18(1):108.
13. Singh JA. The impact of gout on patient's lives: a study of African-American and caucasian men and women with gout. Arthritis Res Ther 2014;16(3):R132.

14. Richardson JC, Liddle J, Mallen CD, et al. Why me? I don't fit the mould ... I am a freak of nature": a qualitative study of women's experience of gout. BMC Womens Health 2015;15:122.

15. Spencer K, Carr A, Doherty M. Patient and provider barriers to effective management of gout in general practice: a qualitative study. Ann Rheum Dis 2012;71(9): 1490–5.

16. Singh JA, Bharat A, Khanna D, et al. Racial differences in health-related quality of life and functional ability in patients with gout. Rheumatology (Oxford) 2017;56(1): 103–12.

17. Wells AF, MacDonald PA, Chefo S, et al. African American patients with gout: efficacy and safety of febuxostat vs allopurinol. BMC Musculoskelet Disord 2012; 13:15.

18. Krishnan E, Lienesch D, Kwoh CK. Gout in ambulatory care settings in the United States. J Rheumatol 2008;35(3):498–501.

19. Solomon DH, Avorn J, Levin R, et al. Uric acid lowering therapy: prescribing patterns in a large cohort of older adults. Ann Rheum Dis 2008;67(5):609–13.

20. Singh JA, Yang S, Saag KG. Factors influencing the effectiveness of allopurinol in achieving and sustaining target serum urate in a US veterans administration gout cohort. J Rheumatol 2019;47(3):449–60.

21. Singh JA. Facilitators and barriers to adherence to urate-lowering therapy in African-Americans with gout: a qualitative study. Arthritis Res Ther 2014; 16(2):R82.

22. Gibson T, Waterworth R, Hatfield P, et al. Hyperuricaemia, gout and kidney function in New Zealand Maori men. Br J Rheumatol 1984;23(4):276–82.

23. Simmonds HA, McBride MB, Hatfield PJ, et al. Polynesian women are also at risk for hyperuricaemia and gout because of a genetic defect in renal urate handling. Br J Rheumatol 1994;33(10):932–7.

24. Dalbeth N, Dowell T, Gerard C, et al. Gout in Aotearoa New Zealand: the equity crisis continues in plain sight. N Z Med J 2018;131(1485):8–12.

25. Dalbeth N, House ME, Horne A, et al. The experience and impact of gout in Maori and Pacific people: a prospective observational study. Clin Rheumatol 2013; 32(2):247–51.

26. Tanner C, Boocock J, Stahl EA, et al. Population-specific resequencing associates the ATP-binding cassette subfamily C member 4 gene with gout in New Zealand Maori and Pacific men. Arthritis Rheumatol 2017;69(7):1461–9.

27. Phipps-Green AJ, Merriman ME, Topless R, et al. Twenty-eight loci that influence serum urate levels: analysis of association with gout. Ann Rheum Dis 2016;75(1): 124–30.

28. Dalbeth N, Gow P, Jackson G, et al. Gout in Aotearoa New Zealand: are we going to ignore this for another 3 years? N Z Med J 2016;129(1429):10–3.

29. Jackson G, Dalbeth N, Te Karu L, et al. Variation in gout care in Aotearoa New Zealand: a national analysis of quality markers. N Z Med J 2014;127(1404): 37–47.

30. Lindsay K, Gow P, Vanderpyl J, et al. The experience and impact of living with gout: a study of men with chronic gout using a qualitative grounded theory approach. J Clin Rheumatol 2011;17(1):1–6.

31. Te Karu L, Bryant L, Elley CR. Maori experiences and perceptions of gout and its treatment: a kaupapa Maori qualitative study. J Prim Health Care 2013;5(3): 214–22.

32. Equity of health care for Māori: a framework. Wellington (New Zealand): Ministry of Health; 2014.

33. Duyck SD, Petrie KJ, Dalbeth N. "You don't have to be a drinker to get gout, but it helps": a content analysis of the depiction of gout in popular newspapers. Arthritis Care Res (Hoboken) 2016;68(11):1721–5.

34. Humphrey C, Hulme R, Dalbeth N, et al. A qualitative study to explore health professionals' experience of treating gout: understanding perceived barriers to effective gout management. J Prim Health Care 2016;8(2):149–56.

35. Kleinstauber M, Wolf L, Jones ASK, et al. Internalized and anticipated stigmatization in patients with gout. ACR Open Rheumatol 2020;2(1):11–7.

36. Holland R, McGill NW. Comprehensive dietary education in treated gout patients does not further improve serum urate. Intern Med J 2015;45(2):189–94.

37. Dalbeth N, Reid S, Stamp LK, et al. Making the right thing the easy thing to do: strategies to improve outcomes in gout. Lancet Rheumatol 2019;1(2):e122–31.

38. Stamp LK, Chapman P, Hudson B, et al. The challenges of managing gout in primary care: results of a best-practice audit. Aust J Gen Pract 2019;48(9):631–7.

39. Bulbin D, Denio AE, Berger A, et al. Improved gout outcomes in primary care using a novel disease management program: a pilot study. Arthritis Care Res (Hoboken) 2018;70(11):1679–85.

40. Callear J, Blakey G, Callear A, et al. Gout in primary care: can we improve patient outcomes? BMJ Qual Improv Rep 2017;6(1). u210130.w4918.

41. Doherty M, Jenkins W, Richardson H, et al. Efficacy and cost-effectiveness of nurse-led care involving education and engagement of patients and a treat-to-target urate-lowering strategy versus usual care for gout: a randomised controlled trial. Lancet 2018;392(10156):1403–12.

42. Fields TR, Rifaat A, Yee AMF, et al. Pilot study of a multidisciplinary gout patient education and monitoring program. Semin Arthritis Rheum 2017;46(5):601–8.

43. Goldfien R, Pressman A, Jacobson A, et al. A pharmacist-staffed, virtual gout management clinic for achieving target serum uric acid levels: a randomized clinical trial. Perm J 2016;20(3):15–234.

44. Mikuls TR, Cheetham TC, Levy GD, et al. Adherence and outcomes with urate-lowering therapy: a site-randomized trial. Am J Med 2019;132(3):354–61.

45. Goldfien RD, Ng MS, Yip G, et al. Effectiveness of a pharmacist-based gout care management programme in a large integrated health plan: results from a pilot study. BMJ Open 2014;4(1):e003627.

46. Rolston CJ, Conner TS, Stamp LK, et al. Improving gout education from patients' perspectives: a focus group study of Maori and Pakeha people with gout. J Prim Health Care 2018;10(3):194–200.

47. Treharne GJ, Richardson AC, Neha T, et al. Education preferences of people with gout: exploring differences between indigenous and nonindigenous peoples from rural and urban locations. Arthritis Care Res (Hoboken) 2018;70(2):260–7.

48. Lawrence A, Scott S, Saparelli F, et al. Facilitating equitable prevention and management of gout for Māori in Northland, New Zealand, through a collaborative primary care approach. J Prim Health Care 2019;11(2):117–27.

49. Marmot M, Bell R. Social determinants and non-communicable diseases: time for integrated action. BMJ 2019;364:l251.

50. Curtis E, Jones R, Tipene-Leach D, et al. Why cultural safety rather than cultural competency is required to achieve health equity: a literature review and recommended definition. Int J Equity Health 2019;18(1):174.

51. Becker MA, Schumacher HR Jr, Wortmann RL, et al. Febuxostat compared with allopurinol in patients with hyperuricemia and gout. N Engl J Med 2005;353(23):2450–61.

52. Schumacher HR Jr, Becker MA, Wortmann RL, et al. Effects of febuxostat versus allopurinol and placebo in reducing serum urate in subjects with hyperuricemia and gout: a 28-week, phase III, randomized, double-blind, parallel-group trial. Arthritis Rheum 2008;59(11):1540–8.

53. Becker MA, Schumacher HR, Espinoza LR, et al. The urate-lowering efficacy and safety of febuxostat in the treatment of the hyperuricemia of gout: the CONFIRMS trial. Arthritis Res Ther 2010;12(2):R63.

54. Terkeltaub RA, Furst DE, Bennett K, et al. High versus low dosing of oral colchicine for early acute gout flare: twenty-four-hour outcome of the first multicenter, randomized, double-blind, placebo-controlled, parallel-group, dose-comparison colchicine study. Arthritis Rheum 2010;62(4):1060–8.

55. Sundy JS, Baraf HS, Yood RA, et al. Efficacy and tolerability of pegloticase for the treatment of chronic gout in patients refractory to conventional treatment: two randomized controlled trials. JAMA 2011;306(7):711–20.

56. Saag KG, Fitz-Patrick D, Kopicko J, et al. Lesinurad combined with allopurinol: a randomized, double-blind, placebo-controlled study in gout patients with an inadequate response to standard-of-care allopurinol (a US-based study). Arthritis Rheumatol 2017;69(1):203–12.

57. Bardin T, Keenan RT, Khanna PP, et al. Lesinurad in combination with allopurinol: a randomised, double-blind, placebo-controlled study in patients with gout with inadequate response to standard of care (the multinational CLEAR 2 study). Ann Rheum Dis 2017;76(5):811–20.

58. Dalbeth N, Jones G, Terkeltaub R, et al. Lesinurad, a selective uric acid reabsorption inhibitor, in combination with febuxostat in patients with tophaceous gout: findings of a phase III clinical trial. Arthritis Rheumatol 2017;69(9):1903–13.

59. Tausche AK, Alten R, Dalbeth N, et al. Lesinurad monotherapy in gout patients intolerant to a xanthine oxidase inhibitor: a 6 month phase 3 clinical trial and extension study. Rheumatology (Oxford) 2017;56(12):2170–8.

Racial Disparities in Systemic Sclerosis

Duncan F. Moore, MD*, Virginia D. Steen, MD

KEYWORDS

- Systemic sclerosis • Scleroderma • Race • Ethnicity • Disparities • Outcomes
- Socioeconomic status

KEY POINTS

- African heritage is associated with a higher incidence of systemic sclerosis than reference white populations, and systemic sclerosis patients of African heritage experience a more severe disease course and ultimately higher mortality.
- Data in other racial or ethnic groups are more limited but suggest that patients of Native North American, Hispanic, and East Asian heritage experience a higher prevalence and severity of selected end-organ manifestations.
- Examinations of socioeconomic status in systemic sclerosis suggest that higher wealth and more equitable access to health care services may mitigate increased mortality attributable to a specific ethnic group.

INTRODUCTION

Systemic sclerosis is a rare and highly morbid autoimmune disease characterized by variable degrees of skin fibrosis and dysfunction of the visceral organs. The burden of systemic sclerosis varies by race and ethnicity. Disparities in health are defined as differential outcomes, including higher disease incidence and morbidity and worse survival, within a population of interest relative to the general population.[1] Disparities among racial and ethnic groups have been a focus of much of the systemic sclerosis disparities literature. Race and ethnicity are social constructs of inexact definitions[2] that can indicate a variable degree of shared genetic heritage, customs, and geographic factors among individuals. Race and ethnicity are linked to socioeconomic status (SES), particularly in the United States[3]; thus it is necessary to consider socioeconomic factors in any examination of disparities by race or ethnicity. This article synthesizes the literature regarding racial and ethnic disparities in systemic sclerosis. Given the variable nomenclature and definitions of racial and ethnic groups among the

Division of Rheumatology, Department of Medicine, MedStar Georgetown University Hospital, 3800 Reservoir Road, PHC 3004, Washington, DC 20007, USA
* Corresponding author.
E-mail address: duncan.f.moore@gunet.georgetown.edu
Twitter: DuncanFMoore (D.F.M.)

Rheum Dis Clin N Am 46 (2020) 705–712
https://doi.org/10.1016/j.rdc.2020.07.009
0889-857X/20/© 2020 Elsevier Inc. All rights reserved.
rheumatic.theclinics.com

studies cited in this article, the authors preserve the group-identifying language used in the original studies when discussing specific findings. The increased burden of systemic sclerosis among nonwhite populations accrues from a higher incidence, more severe disease manifestations, and higher functional impairment and disability. Ultimately, this burden culminates in higher mortality.

EVIDENCE OF DISPARITIES
Incidence and Prevalence

The higher burden of systemic sclerosis in nonwhite ethnicities begins with an increased incidence and prevalence. The most extreme example is that of the Choctaw Native Americans of southeastern Oklahoma. The 4-year period prevalence among full-blooded members of this group was 469 cases per 100,000 population, 31 cases per 100,000 population for less-than-full blooded ($P = .0001$), and 9.5 cases per 100,000 population for other non-Choctaw Native Americans in the region.[4] These rates are dramatically higher than rates among American and European white populations (1.2–25.6 cases per 100,000 population) from a prior 1989 estimate.[5] The increased systemic sclerosis prevalence in this Choctaw group is associated with a specific haplotype on chromosome 15q and is thought to be a founder effect from approximately 10 generations prior.[6]

Data in other indigenous populations have been limited. Within Alberta, Canada, no difference was found in overall systemic sclerosis prevalence among First Nations individuals relative to non-First Nations individuals.[7] The authors suggest that reduced access to rheumatologist care among First Nations individuals may lead to underdiagnosis and thus a falsely low prevalence.

Available incidence data from the United States suggests that black or African American patients have a higher incidence and prevalence of systemic sclerosis. A notable 1997 US cohort demonstrated systemic sclerosis incidence of 14.1 cases per million population per year among black women and 12.8 cases per million population per year among white women ($P<.001$).[8] Another US cohort also demonstrated increased age-specific incidence among black women relative to white women.[9] Mayes and colleagues[10] noted an age-adjusted prevalence ratio of 1.15 (95% CI 1.02–1.30) of blacks relative to whites.

Onset

African Americans,[11–14] black patients in the European Scleroderma Trials and Research group (EUSTAR) cohort,[15] and North American Natives[16] experience systemic sclerosis onset significantly earlier than white patients. Asian patients in the EUSTAR cohort also demonstrated earlier systemic sclerosis onset than white patients,[15] although patients of Chinese descent in 1 Canadian center were older at diagnosis than white patients.[17]

Autoantibodies

Ethnic differences in the prevalence of various systemic sclerosis-specific antibodies are distinct and may illustrate a degree of conserved genetic polymorphisms by ethnic group. Such differences do not intrinsically represent a disparity. However, autoantibodies are associated with several disease manifestations, and even mortality:

- Antitopoisomerase I antibody (ATA) (also known as anti-Scl-70) positivity is an independent predictor of decreased lung function[11] and is associated with interstitial lung disease.[18] ATA is more prevalent among African American patients than either white patients[12–14] or white and Hispanic patients.[19] Canadians of Chinese descent are more likely to be ATA positive than those of European descent.[17]

- Anticentromere antibody (ACA) is associated with limited cutaneous systemic sclerosis (lcSSc) and pulmonary arterial hypertension (PAH).[18] ACA is less prevalent among African Americans,[13,14] Afro-Brazilians,[20] and black patients of the EUSTAR cohort[15] relative to white patients. Asians of the EUSTAR cohort also have lower ACA prevalence than white patients.[15]
- Anti-U1RNP antibody is more prevalent among African American patients than white patients[12–14] and among Chinese descent patients than European descent patients.[17] One study demonstrated a higher prevalence of ILD but no increased mortality among anti-U1RNP-positive African American patients relative to white patients.[13]
- Antifibrillarin antibody (AFA) (also known as U3RNP) is more prevalent among African Americans and Afro-Brazilians than white patients.[13,20] AFA is associated with a higher prevalence of PAH.[13] In a pooled international cohort, AFA was more prevalent among North American Natives,[21] and AFA positivity was independently associated with increased mortality in multivariate analysis (hazard ratio [HR] 1.88, 95% confidence interval [CI] 1.19–2.97, P=.007).

End-Organ Manifestations

Diffuse cutaneous disease (dcSSc) subtype is associated with increased mortality.[8] Thus ethnic differences in the prevalence of cutaneous disease subtype are of concern. Higher prevalence of diffuse disease has been demonstrated among black patients[8,12–15] and First Nations patients[22] relative to white patients. In contrast, other North American studies have not demonstrated ethnic differences in subtype distribution.[17,19,23]

Decreased spirometry values, pulmonary fibrosis, and interstitial lung disease (ILD) in systemic sclerosis have been associated with ethnicity. Pulmonary involvement, defined as ILD or pulmonary hypertension (pHTN), was associated with a twofold higher risk of mortality among all patients during follow-up.[8] Black systemic sclerosis patients have lower forced vital capacity (FVC)[11,12,14,15,19] and diffusing capacity of the lungs for carbon monoxide (DLCO)[11,12,19] relative to whites, even when adjusted for the baseline lower lung volumes among healthy black controls. Hispanic patients had similar spirometry values to both white and African American patients.[19] Asian EUSTAR patients had lower spirometry values than white patients.[15] Among patients with dcSSc and ATA, Japanese patients had a greater decline in FVC during follow-up than did white Americans.[24] African American,[13,19,25] Afro-Brazilian,[20] and Canadian Afro-Caribbean[22] patients have a higher prevalence of radiographic evidence of ILD than white patients. Among ATA-positive patients, African Americans have increased prevalence and severity of pulmonary involvement and increased mortality relative to Caucasians.[13] In a study by Kuwana and colleagues,[24] black, Choctaw Native American, and Japanese patients all had higher prevalence of radiographic ILD than white patients. pHTN is also more prevalent among African American[8,14] and Afro-Brazilian[20] patients than white patients, although this is likely secondary to in part the higher prevalence of ILD.

Severe digital symptoms and calcinosis vary in prevalence by ethnicity. Black patients have had higher rates of pitting,[12,25] digital ulcerations,[12] digital infarcts,[8] and digital ischemia (pitting, ulcers, or gangrene)[14] than white patients. In contrast, one US cohort showed no racial difference in severe skin disease (ulcers or gangrene).[13] North American Asian patients have been shown to have fewer digital ulcerations[17,23] and lower prevalence of calcinosis than white or Caucasian patients.[22]

Myositis in systemic sclerosis patients is more frequent among black or African Americans[8,13] and Chinese Canadians[17] than whites. Of note, myositis is more common in diffuse disease.[8]

Gastrointestinal (GI) manifestations, particularly small bowel involvement, are more frequent among African American than Caucasian systemic sclerosis patients[13] and among African American and Hispanic patients than white patients.[19] However, no such ethnic difference was demonstrated in 2 other studies.[14,25] North American Native ethnicity is associated with increased GI symptoms relative to white ethnicity.[16] East Asians had less esophageal dysmotility than patients of European descent.[22]

Functional Impairment, Quality of Life, and Disability

In the Genetics versus Environment in Scleroderma Outcome Study (GENISOS) cohort, white patients were noted to have higher (better) scores on the physical component summary of the 36-Item Short Form Survey (SF-36) and lower Scleroderma-HAQ scores (indicating better physical ability) than African American or Hispanic patients.[26] Analysis by Steen and colleagues[13] of a Pittsburgh cohort noted increased HAQ disability index scores at the index visit among African Americans relative to Caucasian patients. This was thought to be caused by a higher prevalence of dcSSc among the African Americans. In a pooled analysis of dcSSc patients, Hispanic patients had a higher (more severe) patient global assessment of disease severity than both African American and Caucasian patients,[27] but no differences in physician global assessment scores. This discrepancy in patient- and physician-assessed disease severity could possibly reflect some combination of ethnic difference in disease perception or under-recognition by the examiners of severity in Hispanic patients.

Analysis of the GENISOS cohort demonstrated that, at enrollment, ethnicity did not correlate with work disability, but decreased educational attainment and reduced social support did.[28] It is hypothesized that patients with lower educational attainment are more likely to have a physically demanding job with which the progressive disability of systemic sclerosis will more quickly yield work disability. Notably, as the course progressed, nonwhite ethnicity was noted to be an independent predictor of work disability at follow-up.

Treatment

Studies have not demonstrated ethnic group differences in immunomodulatory drug use in systemic sclerosis[17,23,25] with the exception of higher corticosteroid use at any point among African Americans[25] and among patients of Chinese descent[17] relative to reference populations. Higher corticosteroid use likely is attributable to the higher prevalence of myositis within these groups. Within, but particularly outside of a universal health care system, it remains plausible that the real-world, nontrial adherence to immunosuppressive regimens by systemic sclerosis patients may be reduced among patients of lower SES due to treatment cost and other barriers.

Mortality

Across the entirety of the United States, the age-adjusted mortality rate secondary to systemic sclerosis is 7.1 cases per 1 million population in black patients, 4.4 cases per 1 million population in white patients, and 3.0 cases per 1 million population in patients of other races.[29] However, these differential mortality rates by race do not account for racial differences in systemic sclerosis incidence.

Within systemic sclerosis cohorts throughout the world, it is clear that black race or African heritage, unadjusted, is a risk factor for increased mortality during follow-up.

Meta-analysis of 5 cohorts revealed that African origin is associated in univariate survival analysis with an HR of death of 1.38 (95% CI 1.15–1.66).[30] Within US cohorts, black patients had approximately twofold higher unadjusted mortality[13,14,25] and 1.6- to twofold higher age-adjusted mortality[8,14] than white populations. Other US multivariate survival analyses that demonstrated increased mortality among black systemic sclerosis patients included: (1) adjustment for age, sex, and diffuse disease status[13] and (2) adjustment for sex, disease duration, diffuse disease status, and either systemic sclerosis-specific autoantibody status, educational attainment, or health insurance type.[14] A cohort composed of American and Japanese patients with systemic sclerosis and ATA demonstrated increased mortality among both Japanese and African American patients relative to white American patients.[24]

African heritage has also been associated with increased mortality outside of the United States. Afro-Brazilians had higher mortality than white Brazilians, even when adjusted for age, gender, and diffuse disease status.[20]

The international EUSTAR cohort, which includes centers in China and South Africa, also demonstrated higher unadjusted mortality risks among Asian and black patients relative to white patients.[15] However, in individual-matched mortality analyses (in which patients of different races were matched 1:1 for age, sex, diffuse skin disease status, and disease duration), these mortality differences by ethnicity were no longer statistically significant.

In a multivariate survival analysis (sex, ethnicity, age at enrollment, treatment site) of a pooled cohort of American, Canadian, and Australian patients, African descent was associated with increased mortality (HR 2.05, 95% CI 1.25–3.36, $P = .005$), as was Australian Aboriginal ethnicity (HR 15.78, 95% CI 2.15–115.58, $P=.007$).[21]

However, the aforementioned mortality evaluations by race or ethnicity largely did not account for SES. Socioeconomic factors that correlate with race, particularly within the United States, may represent effect modifiers, interaction (ie, synergistic) terms, or mediating factors in the assessment of the independent mortality effect. Within the systemic sclerosis literature, black patients have been shown to have less educational attainment[12,25,31] and decreased household income[25,31] relative to nonblack patients. North American Natives with systemic sclerosis have also been shown to have lower educational attainment and income and are more likely to live in a rural residence than white systemic sclerosis patients.[16] In the GENISOS cohort, nonwhite patients have lower household income and less access to private transportation.[32] SES covariates that have been used in systemic sclerosis mortality research include marital status, employment, educational attainment, insurance status, and household income.[14,25,31] In a recent single-center US cohort, following multivariate adjustment for these aforementioned socioeconomic factors, African American race was not an independent risk factor for increased mortality during follow-up; however, decreased imputed income was independently associated with a higher risk of death during follow-up, independent of race.[25] For every additional $10,000 in household income, the hazard of death during follow-up decreased by 15.5%.

In contrast, there are recent studies in nations with universal health care, including Canada[22] and France,[30] that do not demonstrate survival differences among patients of Afro-Caribbean or African origin, respectively, relative to patients of European descent. This suggests that more equitable access to care may blunt any mortality effects inherent in African heritage. In fact, the Canadian study demonstrated that all ethnic groups examined (European-descent white, Afro-Caribbean, South Asian, East Asian, Hispanic, and First Nations) had similar survival per a multivariate Cox regression adjusted for age, era of treatment, and comorbidities.[22] Analysis of a separate Canadian cohort noted that decreased educational attainment, a proxy for lower SES, did not correlate with mortality during follow-up.[33]

SUMMARY

Racial and ethnic disparities in systemic sclerosis are abundant. Patients of African heritage experience higher incidence, earlier onset, more end-organ disease, lower quality of life, and higher mortality than reference populations. Remarkably, despite differences in disease incidence and manifestations that have a degree of genetic underpinning, strong evidence exists that black patients experience similar mortality as reference populations when they experience similar SES or suffer in the setting of a universal health care system. Data on indigenous peoples are sparse, but notably a Choctaw group from Oklahoma have experienced higher incidence of systemic sclerosis and more ILD likely because of a founder effect. Other data suggest (Canadian) North American Natives experience worse GI symptoms. Relative data in Hispanic patients are also limited but suggest they experience higher prevalence of ILD and GI symptoms and lower quality of life. Asian populations have been shown to have worse lung function and more prevalent ILD and myositis but better digital symptoms than reference populations.

Individually, each report of disparity can be diminished by honing in on the numerous measured and unmeasured interacting and modifying factors, such as household income, inherent in a predominantly retrospective disparities literature in this rare disease. In aggregate, the trends cannot be discounted. Moving forward, whether in international systemic sclerosis registries, treatment trials, or at a genomic level, researchers must continue to characterize racial and ethnic disparities in systemic sclerosis and continue to situate them in their more local and modifiable socioeconomic contexts.

DISCLOSURE

The authors have nothing to disclose.

REFERENCES

1. Alvidrez J, Castille D, Laude-Sharp M, et al. The National Institute on Minority Health and Health Disparities Research Framework. Am J Public Health 2019; 109(S1):S16–20.
2. Witzig R. The medicalization of race: scientific legitimization of a flawed social construct. Ann Intern Med 1996;125(8):675–9.
3. Kaufman JS, Cooper RS, McGee DL. Socioeconomic status and health in blacks and whites: the problem of residual confounding and the resiliency of race. Epidemiology 1997;8(6):621–8.
4. Arnett FC, Howard RF, Tan F, et al. Increased prevalence of systemic sclerosis in a Native American tribe in Oklahoma. Association with an Amerindian HLA haplotype. Arthritis Rheum 1996;39(8):1362–70.
5. Lawrence RC, Hochberg MC, Kelsey JL, et al. Estimates of the prevalence of selected arthritic and musculoskeletal diseases in the United States. J Rheumatol 1989;16(4):427–41.
6. Tan FK, Stivers DN, Foster MW, et al. Association of microsatellite markers near the fibrillin 1 gene on human chromosome 15q with scleroderma in a Native American population. Arthritis Rheum 1998;41(10):1729–37.

7. Barnabe C, Joseph L, Belisle P, et al. Prevalence of systemic lupus erythematosus and systemic sclerosis in the First Nations population of Alberta, Canada. Arthritis Care Res (Hoboken) 2012;64(1):138–43.

8. Laing TJ, Gillespie BW, Toth MB, et al. Racial differences in scleroderma among women in Michigan. Arthritis Rheum 1997;40(4):734–42.

9. Steen VD, Oddis CV, Conte CG, et al. Incidence of systemic sclerosis in Allegheny County, Pennsylvania. A twenty-year study of hospital-diagnosed cases, 1963-1982. Arthritis Rheum 1997;40(3):441–5.

10. Mayes MD, Lacey JV, Beebe-Dimmer J, et al. Prevalence, incidence, survival, and disease characteristics of systemic sclerosis in a large US population. Arthritis Rheum 2003;48(8):2246–55.

11. Greidinger EL, Flaherty KT, White B, et al. African-American race and antibodies to topoisomerase I are associated with increased severity of scleroderma lung disease. Chest 1998;114(3):801–7.

12. Nietert PJ, Mitchell HC, Bolster MB, et al. Racial variation in clinical and immunological manifestations of systemic sclerosis. J Rheumatol 2006;33(2):263–8.

13. Steen V, Domsic RT, Lucas M, et al. A clinical and serologic comparison of African American and Caucasian patients with systemic sclerosis. Arthritis Rheum 2012; 64(9):2986–94.

14. Gelber AC, Manno RL, Shah AA, et al. Race and association with disease manifestations and mortality in scleroderma: a 20-year experience at the Johns Hopkins Scleroderma Center and review of the literature. Medicine (Baltimore) 2013; 92(4):191–205.

15. Jaeger VK, Tikly M, Xu D, et al. Racial differences in systemic sclerosis disease presentation: a European Scleroderma Trials and Research group study. Rheumatology (Oxford) 2019. https://doi.org/10.1093/rheumatology/kez486.

16. Bacher A, Mittoo S, Hudson M, et al. Systemic sclerosis in Canada's North American Native population: assessment of clinical and serological manifestations. J Rheumatol 2013;40(7):1121–6.

17. Low AHL, Johnson SR, Lee P. Ethnic influence on disease manifestations and autoantibodies in Chinese-descent patients with systemic sclerosis. J Rheumatol 2009;36(4):787–93.

18. Steen VD. The many faces of scleroderma. Rheum Dis Clin North Am 2008;34(1): 1–15, v.

19. McNearney TA, Reveille JD, Fischbach M, et al. Pulmonary involvement in systemic sclerosis: associations with genetic, serologic, sociodemographic, and behavioral factors. Arthritis Rheum 2007;57(2):318–26.

20. Mendes C, Viana VST, Pasoto SG, et al. Clinical and laboratory features of African-Brazilian patients with systemic sclerosis. Clin Rheumatol 2020; 39(1):9–17.

21. Mejia Otero C, Assassi S, Hudson M, et al. Antifibrillarin antibodies are associated with native North American ethnicity and poorer survival in systemic sclerosis. J Rheumatol 2017;44(6):799–805.

22. Al-Sheikh H, Ahmad Z, Johnson SR. Ethnic variations in systemic sclerosis disease manifestations, internal organ involvement, and mortality. J Rheumatol 2019. https://doi.org/10.3899/jrheum.180042.

23. Schmajuk G, Bush TM, Burkham J, et al. Characterizing systemic sclerosis in Northern California: focus on Asian and Hispanic patients. Clin Exp Rheumatol 2009;27(3 Suppl 54):22–5.

24. Kuwana M, Kaburaki J, Arnett FC, et al. Influence of ethnic background on clinical and serologic features in patients with systemic sclerosis and anti-DNA topoisomerase I antibody. Arthritis Rheum 1999;42(3):465–74.

25. Moore DF, Kramer E, Eltaraboulsi R, et al. Increased morbidity and mortality of scleroderma in African Americans compared to non-African Americans. Arthritis Care Res (Hoboken) 2019. https://doi.org/10.1002/acr.23861.

26. McNearney TA, Hunnicutt SE, Fischbach M, et al. Perceived functioning has ethnic-specific associations in systemic sclerosis: another dimension of personalized medicine. J Rheumatol 2009;36(12):2724–32.

27. Nashid M, Khanna PP, Furst DE, et al. Gender and ethnicity differences in patients with diffuse systemic sclerosis–analysis from three large randomized clinical trials. Rheumatology (Oxford) 2011;50(2):335–42.

28. Sharif R, Mayes MD, Nicassio PM, et al. Determinants of work disability in patients with systemic sclerosis: a longitudinal study of the GENISOS cohort. Semin Arthritis Rheum 2011;41(1):38–47.

29. Mendoza F, Derk CT. Systemic sclerosis mortality in the United States: 1999-2002 implications for patient care. J Clin Rheumatol 2007;13(4):187–92.

30. Pokeerbux MR, Giovannelli J, Dauchet L, et al. Survival and prognosis factors in systemic sclerosis: data of a French multicenter cohort, systematic review, and meta-analysis of the literature. Arthritis Res Ther 2019;21(1):86.

31. Nietert PJ, Silver RM, Mitchell HC, et al. Demographic and clinical factors associated with in-hospital death among patients with systemic sclerosis. J Rheumatol 2005;32(10):1888–92.

32. Reveille JD, Fischbach M, McNearney T, et al. Systemic sclerosis in 3 US ethnic groups: a comparison of clinical, sociodemographic, serologic, and immunogenetic determinants. Semin Arthritis Rheum 2001;30(5):332–46.

33. Mansour S, Bonner A, Muangchan C, et al. Low socioeconomic status (measured by education) and outcomes in systemic sclerosis: data from the Canadian Scleroderma Research Group. J Rheumatol 2013;40(4):447–54.

III. Strategies to Begin to Reduce Disparities

Increasing Ancestral Diversity in Lupus Trials

Ways Forward

Titilola Falasinnu, PhD[a,b,]*, Yashaar Chaichian, MD[c,1],
Julia F. Simard, ScD[a,d]

KEYWORDS

- Diversity • Clinical trials • Lupus • Biomedical studies • Health disparities
- Heterogeneity • Treatment response

KEY POINTS

- One important means of addressing disparities is to ensure that the inclusion of race/ethnic minorities in systemic lupus erythematosus (SLE) clinical trials is adequate.
- There are many indications that treatment response in SLE may be heterogeneous by race/ethnicity based on our understanding of the epidemiology of the disease.
- We recommend that clinical trials in SLE move beyond *only* increasing race/ethnic diversity to ensuring adequately powered subgroup analyses.
- Diversity efforts should also be focused on biomedical studies to ensure that the pathophysiology of race/ethnic minorities are adequately represented.
- We present a framework for improving generalizability of clinical research in SLE through patient-, clinician-, and institutional-level engagements across the research continuum.

INTRODUCTION

Biomedical and clinical research can have a major impact on the eradication of health disparities, which unfortunately remain common among a wide range of chronic conditions.[1–3] There is a significant need to address disparities in systemic lupus erythematosus (SLE), and this is increasingly recognized within the SLE research and clinical community as a research priority.[4–7] There are different ways to address this issue. One important means is to ensure that the inclusion of race/ethnic minorities in SLE

^a Department of Epidemiology and Population Health, Stanford Medicine, 150 Governor's Lane, Stanford, CA, USA; ^b Department of Anesthesiology, Perioperative, and Pain Medicine, Stanford Medicine, 150 Governor's Lane, Stanford, CA, USA; ^c Division of Immunology and Rheumatology, Department of Medicine, Stanford Medicine, Stanford, CA, USA; ^d Division of Immunology and Rheumatology, Department of Medicine, Stanford Medicine, 150 Governor's Lane, Stanford, CA, USA
¹ Present address: 900 Blake Wilbur Drive W2081, Palo Alto, CA 94304.
* Corresponding author. 150 Governor's Lane, Stanford, CA.
E-mail address: tof@stanford.edu

Rheum Dis Clin N Am 46 (2020) 713–722
https://doi.org/10.1016/j.rdc.2020.07.011
0889-857X/20/© 2020 Elsevier Inc. All rights reserved.

rheumatic.theclinics.com

clinical trials is adequate. In a review of 193 clinical trials for SLE with at least 1 site in the United States, we found that although race/ethnic minorities comprise nearly 70% of estimated prevalent SLE cases (43% Black, 16% Hispanic, and 13% Asian), they comprise only 49% of clinical trial participants (14% Black, 21% Hispanic, and 10% Asian).[8] The study also found that the representation of Black individuals among trial enrollees has decreased since 2006 to 2011, whereas the representation of other race/ ethnic minorities has increased.[8] However, the lack of diversity in clinical trials is not unique to SLE.[9] To provide a broader context, we draw extensively from oncology where the issue of diversity in clinical trials has a long history, and we highlight parallels to SLE. We recommend that clinical trials in SLE move beyond *only* increasing race/ ethnic diversity to ensuring adequately powered subgroup analyses due to the pre- ponderance of evidence for race/ethnic differences in response to therapeutic agents in SLE. In this article, we further argue that focusing diversity efforts on clinical trial recruitment alone is insufficient because this ignores decision-making that occurs up- stream and downstream of clinical trials that may adversely impact these efforts. We present a framework (**Fig. 1**) for improving generalizability of clinical research in SLE through patient-level, clinician-level, and institutional-level engagements across the research continuum.

HISTORICAL AND CONTEMPORARY TRENDS REGARDING DIVERSITY IN CLINICAL TRIALS

In the United States, the problem of lack of race/ethnic diversity is multidimensional, shaped by social determinants of health. This also limits the generalizability of trial re- sults and can have unintended consequences, such as preventing minorities from adequately benefiting from scientific advances stemming from clinical trials. In addi- tion to our finding of the underrepresentation of race/ethnic minorities in SLE random- ized controlled trials (RCTs), ample evidence exists for this in other medical subspecialties. In an attempt to quantify the generalizability of trials for the US popu- lation, Loree and colleagues[10] reported on the following mismatch: between the

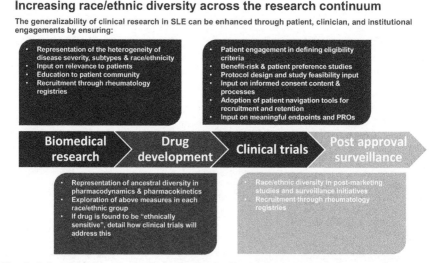

Fig. 1. Enhancing diversity in the research pipeline: a democratizing framework.

proportion of different races represented in trials for US Food and Drug Administration (FDA) approval of oncology drugs for specific indications with the proportion of different races (pertaining to incidence and mortality) among patients with a specific type of cancer versus the US population. There was consistent underrepresentation of Black and Hispanic patients in pivotal FDA approval studies between July 2008 and June 2018, with White, Asian, Black, and Hispanic patients representing 76%, 18%, 3%, and 6% of trial enrollees in oncology, respectively.[10] Similar to our findings in SLE RCTs, Loree and colleagues[10] found that the proportion of Black enrollees decreased or stayed the same over time (4% to 3% between 2008 and 2018), suggesting that this decline in representation may not be unique to SLE.

We highlight a few key time points in the modern era in which national policies for increasing the reporting and representation of race/ethnic minorities in clinical trials have implications for SLE. In 1993, the National Institutes of Health (NIH) Revitalization Act stated that women and minorities must be included in all NIH-funded clinical research, unless there is a justification approved by the NIH.[11,12] An amendment was issued by the NIH in 2001 mandating that proposals for NIH-defined phase III clinical trials define processes for identifying differences in treatment responses among race/ethnic groups if the intervention effect is expected to differ among them.[11,12] In 2017, NIH issued a policy revision requiring that applicable NIH-defined phase III clinical trials submit subgroup analyses by race/ethnicity and sex/gender to Clinicaltrials.gov.[11,12] In 2018, Geller and colleagues[13] published a review to investigate the contemporary levels of compliance with these guidelines in NIH-funded RCTs published in 14 leading US medical journals. They found that 85% of the published RCTs did not include race/ethnicity in the analysis and did not provide an explanation for this exclusion.[13] When they compared this finding with their previous examination of these trends in 2004, 2009, and 2015, they found no statistically significant improvements in the lack of compliance with the guidelines between 2004 and 2018.[13]

DOES TREATMENT RESPONSE VARY BY RACE/ETHNICITY IN SYSTEMIC LUPUS ERYTHEMATOSUS?

Although there have certainly been advances in the treatment of SLE in the past decade, the therapeutic landscape has not changed as rapidly as hoped. Hydroxychloroquine remains the cornerstone of treatment, with glucocorticoids used for flares (with a goal to taper to a low dose as soon as is feasible), along with various immunosuppressive agents that are used to induce and maintain remission, as well as facilitate steroid taper.[14] Cyclophosphamide is used for severe SLE manifestations when other agents are not appropriate, as well as in refractory disease, a setting in which rituximab also can play a role.[14] Despite increased understanding of disease pathogenesis, most SLE clinical trials of new targeted therapies have failed.[15] One exception is belimumab, which is currently approved for use in patients with active, nonrenal, non–central nervous system SLE.[16] Several other drugs have shown promise in recent clinical trials, although are not yet approved therapies.[17–22]

Our review did not ascertain whether SLE RCTs provided subgroup analyses by race/ethnicity in accordance with the NIH policy; however, there are many indications that treatment response in SLE may be heterogeneous by race/ethnicity based on our understanding of the epidemiology of the disease. Here, we present several mechanistic bases for race/ethnic differences in response to therapeutic agents in SLE. First, race/ethnic minorities share a disproportionate burden in risk of SLE, and the immunologic profile, clinical presentation, and overall prognosis differ by race/ethnicity.[23] There are also differences in the immunologic profiles (in particular autoantibodies) by race/ethnicity. There are no reported race/ethnic differences in antinuclear antibody, although Black patients with SLE are known to have higher prevalence of positivity for specific autoantibodies, such as anti-Sm, anti-RNP and anti-dsDNA, compared with White patients.[24] Taken together, these race/ethnic differences in SLE phenotypes suggest possible race/ethnic-dependent biological pathways that underlie the expression of disease.

Second, these disparities are also evident in mortality, where the rates are highest in Black individuals, followed by Hispanic and White individuals. SLE is also a significant cause of premature mortality for women of reproductive age. A recent study of death certificate data in the United States found that SLE was the fifth leading cause of death in Black and Hispanic 15-year-old to 24-year-old female patients, behind neoplasms, heart disease, infections, and pregnancy, a remarkable finding given that SLE is defined as a rare disease.[25] Third, in a study of major treatment advancements in the context of SLE mortality rates, Singh and Yen[26] found significant declines in mortality since the 1950s attributed to the improving understanding of the pathophysiology of the disease and advancements in treatment options. There are indications that race/ethnic minorities may have not fully benefited from these therapeutic advances.[27]

Fourth, one question that emerges from these disparities in mortality is whether these differences could be attributed to biological, genetic, environmental, and/or socioeconomic determinants. Although it could be argued that it might be more useful to infer genetic ancestry ascertaining (eg, through genome-wide association studies [GWAS]) instead of using race/ethnicity in understanding the pathophysiology of disease, this issue is complicated because both constructs capture different information.[28] However, complex traits, and polygenic and environmental factors may be shaped by ancestry and social determinants of health.[28] A major possible contributory factor is that the current treatment options for SLE may not be as appropriate for race/ethnic minorities and treatment guidelines are not optimized to address this issue. However, comparing studies that report differences in treatment response can be difficult due to differences in measurement and the changing nature of race/ethnic identity.[23] Also, most studies showing differences in treatment response are often underpowered in post hoc analyses.[23]

There have been little to no "head-to-head" comparisons by race/ethnicity of heterogeneity in SLE treatment response in observational or experimental settings. In a review evaluating the evidence for race differences in the response to therapies for SLE, Litwic and colleagues[23] reported that there are no major race/ethnic differences in the response to steroids, hydroxychloroquine, and azathioprine. However, this conclusion can be misleading because there have been no biomedical or clinical research studies evaluating whether there are differences in response to these medications by race/ethnicity. Future studies are needed to answer this question. Among therapeutic agents for induction therapy for lupus nephritis, intravenous cyclophosphamide (IVC) may be less effective in Black and Hispanic patients compared with White patients.[29,30] For example, Dooley and colleagues[29] reported that the 5-year renal survival for patients on IVC was 95% in non-Black patients, whereas it was 57% in Black patients. Mycophenolate mofetil for lupus nephritis appears to be more effective in Black and Hispanic patients compared with White patients.[23,30] There is also some indication that mycophenolate mofetil is safer and causes fewer side effects in these groups.[23,30,31] However, there are significant methodologic limitations to these studies, including sample size and reference groups (that include all non-Black patients) that limit the generalizability of their inferences.

HETEROGENEITY IN SYSTEMIC LUPUS ERYTHEMATOSUS AND THE CHALLENGE OF CLINICAL TRIALS AND BIOMEDICAL STUDIES

The heterogeneity of SLE presents a unique set of challenges in clinical trials and biomedical studies. For example, there are differences in the association of SLE with genetic factors by race/ethnicity. One recent GWAS identified 58 distinct non-HLA regions in White, 9 in Black, and 16 in Hispanic individuals.[32] There was a lack of considerable overlap in the genetic regions by race/ethnicity.[32] When evaluating how well the "White"-associated genetic factors predicted SLE, the odds ratio was 30, but when applied to the Black population the odds ratio was only 3, highlighting the differences in genetic association by race/ethnicity in SLE.[32,33] In clinical trials, this heterogeneity leads to smaller, mostly homogeneous cohorts that often do not adequately represent the broad spectrum of the disease. In biomedical and biomarker studies, this challenge may be reflected in the lack of understanding of more severe and less prevalent subtypes. This issue is particularly important because one of the biggest benefits of "-omics" and biomarkers research is the possibility of discovering novel pathobiological pathways.[34] Biomarkers discovered in homogeneous cohorts may only generalize to external cohorts similar to the original cohort and may be less useful in a cohort that differs significantly from the original cohort.[34] Conversely, biomarkers discovered using heterogeneous cohorts may be more likely to generalize to a more comprehensive spectrum of disease subtypes.[34] The proliferation of GWAS has been useful in discovering significant associations between genetic variants and biological traits. However, only 3% of the participants in the National Human Genome Research Institute GWAS catalog (the most comprehensive publicly available resource of human genetic association research) are of African ancestry.[28] Although our review found a lack of representation of race/ethnic minorities in RCTs of patients with SLE, much is unknown about whether biomedical studies take advantage of the rich ancestral diversity of patients with SLE. Specifically, how representative of the spectrum of disease severity and subtypes are the samples/specimens used to develop biomarkers for SLE?

Examples of the consequences of the lack of diversity in biomedical studies are ample. For example, the first iteration of the human papillomavirus (HPV) vaccine covered 2 subtypes of the infection, however, Black women are 50% less likely to have HPV subtypes represented in those vaccines.[35,36] Although the newest versions of the vaccines now protect against 9 HPV subtypes, the most common HPV subtypes found in Black women are still not covered by these new iterations of the vaccines.[35] As a corollary, the identification and characterization of the molecular biological pathways distinctively driving refractory manifestations in racially and ethnically diverse populations that lead to higher mortality in minority groups have yet to be established in SLE. This means that the development of therapeutic agents that are more suitable for the phenotypes in race/ethnic minorities may be delayed. Future studies in these directions are warranted to develop clinically applicable preventive and therapeutic strategies for better SLE management.

The pharmacogenetic differences in the frequencies of variants associated with drug metabolism may translate to certain therapeutic agents being safer and more efficacious in some race/ethnic groups than others. For example, the CYP2D6 gene is responsible for the metabolism and elimination of 25% of commonly prescribed drugs.[28] Race is a major determinant of variability in the CYP2D6 gene.[28] Several GWAS have identified associations between treatment responses and clinically relevant genetic variants.[28] The lack of efficacy of cyclophosphamide in Black patients with SLE may be due to the twofold higher level of toxic metabolites of this agent in

Black patients compared with White patients.[23] This issue is also reflected in the high rates of adverse events in clinical trials of cyclophosphamide in Black patients.[23] Despite these findings, there is a surprising lack of evidence of the race/ethnic composition of drug development studies for SLE. The consequences of knowing little about the pharmacogenomics, pharmacodynamics, and pharmacokinetics of SLE drugs in race/ethnic minorities may translate to less effective (or in some cases, potentially harmful) dosage decisions for these populations. This may also lead to issues with medication adherence in race/ethnic minorities. If there is heterogeneity in pharmacodynamics and pharmacokinetics by race/ethnicity, efforts should be made to address this issue before planning the RCTs (see **Fig. 1**).

In 2019, the FDA issued draft guidelines to broaden clinical trials eligibility criteria and avoid unnecessary exclusions by improving recruitment for trial participants to reflect the population likely to use the drug.[9] The inclusive practices recommendations include accounting for the serologic and immunologic markers before excluding patients with human immunodeficiency virus, hepatitis, and tuberculosis, and noted that patients can be stable on medication used to treat these underlying conditions and still be eligible for clinical trials.[9] The guidelines also requested that trialists use evidence-based exclusions to limit the participation of individuals with renal, cardiac, and hepatic function and recommended that clinical trials include patients with mild organ dysfunction, for example.[9] These recommendations may be useful for clinical trials in SLE in which eligibility may, in some cases, be considered stringent. In a study of the eligibility of lupus nephritis trials, Collinson and colleagues[37] applied published trial eligibility criteria to a large registry of patients with SLE in the United Kingdom. They found that 51% of the registry did not satisfy the inclusion and exclusion criteria, making them ineligible for study entry.[37] The extent to which this finding varies by race/ethnicity is unknown; however, overly stringent inclusion/exclusion criteria may have significant implications for the study of treatment options in more severe disease and in race/ethnic minorities.

ENHANCING DIVERSITY IN THE SYSTEMIC LUPUS ERYTHEMATOSUS RESEARCH PIPELINE: A DEMOCRATIZING FRAMEWORK

In this section, we propose potential solutions to the barriers to diversifying the research pipeline for SLE drugs identified in the previous section. The lack of diversity in biomedical and clinical trial research may be related to both provider and patient-related factors. Clinician-focused interventions should include increasing awareness and knowledge, addressing implicit bias (where present), and removing logistical hindrances.[38] For example, some providers may have limited knowledge of available clinical trials and they may also have beliefs that race/ethnic minorities may not understand or adhere to trial protocols.[38] Other barriers to recruiting race/ethnic minorities include limited time to talk to patients during their consultations and limited clinical trial sites within close proximity to the provider's practice location.[38] Finally, clinician communication may not be culturally and linguistically tailored to understanding the needs of the patients in their practice. To be clear, these are provider barriers that exist throughout medicine, and are not unique to rheumatologists. Nevertheless, to address these challenges, the American College of Rheumatology (ACR) developed Materials to Increase Minority Involvement in Clinical Trials (MIMICT), an education program for clinicians involved in SLE care. MIMICT connects clinical trial sites and clinicians to provide resources for discussing clinical trial opportunities with patients.[38] Another ACR initiative, Lupus Clinical Trials Training (LuCTT), is a didactic program that aims to increase community health workers' knowledge and skills to educate and support Black and Hispanic patients with SLE in navigating clinical trials and the health care system.[38]

Race/ethnic minorities may have limited access to clinicians involved in clinical trials. Patient-level barriers to participating in clinical trials include lack of access, opportunity, mistrust, health literacy, and cultural factors.[38] Other access issues include lack of health insurance, lack of transportation to trial sites, frequency of blood draws, extra office visits, restrictive child care options, and inability to miss work.[38] In addition, the historical exploitation of the Black community in clinical and biomedical research may have a lingering effect on recruitment of these patients into clinical trials.[38–41] This may be attributed to medical mistrust and could be mitigated by having a more diverse clinical trials workforce, as only approximately 1% of rheumatologists in the United States are Black.[42] Evidence suggests that racial concordance between doctor and patient matter for the utilization of preventive medicine.[43]

In the framework presented in this article, we highlight ways in which patient/community education and engagement needs to be prioritized when designing biomedical studies and interventions. Patient groups should be engaged across the research continuum: from formulating research areas that are relevant to patients to providing input on meaningful endpoints and patient-reported outcomes. To overcome patient-level barriers related to costs and logistics, efforts to recruit and retain race/ethnic minorities in RCTs may require labor-intensive measures and culturally appropriate and more personal contacts. One such initiative is patient navigation or the use of lay community health workers to educate patients about RCTs and provide individualized support for patients enrolled in these clinical trials.[44] A study that evaluated the adoption of patient navigators for the recruitment and retention of Black patients in clinical trials at a cancer center in the United States found that 75% of patients receiving patient navigation support completed the RCT compared with 38% of patients without this intervention.[44] Based on this compelling evidence, future studies should consider adopting the patient navigation model for SLE RCTs. In terms of institutional-level removal of barriers to race/ethnic minorities enrolling in RCTs, we suggest that NIH incentivize efforts to diversify RCTs to encourage trial sites to comply with current guidelines. Finally, to diversify the sampling frame for biomedical and clinical research, disease registries have been used to identify trial participants for multicenter RCTs, trials involving rare diseases or race/ethnic minorities.[45] Trialists may consider querying the Rheumatology Informatics System for Effectiveness (RISE) Registry using inclusion/exclusion criteria to facilitate recruitment, thus democratizing the process and increasing efficiency and the probability of success.

SUMMARY

Significant disparities exist in SLE regarding prevalence, disease severity, and mortality, with race/ethnic minorities being disproportionately affected. Despite these disparities, race/ethnic minorities are underrepresented within SLE research, whether basic science-related (eg, GWAS) or in the recruitment of patients for clinical trials of new therapeutic agents. Both provider and patient-related barriers to their participation likely play a role. Decreased race/ethnic minority involvement in SLE research has real-world implications, including less understanding of the disease itself and less applicability of approved therapies among this group of patients. Although the underrepresentation of race/ethnic minorities and barriers to their participation in research are not unique to SLE, members of the lupus research community have an obligation to narrow this gap going forward to ensure that future advances within the field are derived from and benefit a more representative group of patients.

DISCLOSURE

Y. Chaichian has received support from Gilead Sciences, AMPEL BioSolutions, Pfizer, GSK, and the Lupus Research Alliance. The other authors have nothing to disclose.

REFERENCES

1. Sue S, Dhindsa MK. Ethnic and racial health disparities research: issues and problems. Health Educ Behav 2006;33(4):459–69.
2. Centers for Disease Control and Prevention. Special feature on racial and ethnic health disparities. Heal United States. 2015;3:216. Available at: https://www.cdc.gov/nchs/data/hus/hus15.pdf.
3. 2015 National Healthcare Quality and Disparities Report and 5th Anniversary Update on the National Quality Strategy | Agency for Health Research and Quality. Available at: https://www.ahrq.gov/research/findings/nhqrdr/nhqdr15/index.html. Accessed March 11, 2020.
4. Arntsen KA, Raymond SC, Farber KM. Lupus: Patient Voices Report on Externally-Led Patient-Focused Drug Development Meeting A Message of Gratitude. Available at: http://www.lupuspfdd.org/LupusPatientVoicesFINAL.pdf.
5. To bridge health disparities, diagnose lupus early & improve access - the rheumatologist. Available at: https://www.the-rheumatologist.org/article/to-bridge-health-disparities-diagnose-lupus-early-improve-access/?singlepage=1&theme=print-friendly. Accessed March 11, 2020.
6. Lupus Highlighted in New Congressional Report on Health Disparities | Lupus Foundation of America. Available at: https://www.lupus.org/news/lupus-highlighted-in-new-congressional-report-on-health-disparities. Accessed March 11, 2020.
7. Lupus Grants - The Office of Minority Health. Available at: https://minorityhealth.hhs.gov/omh/browse.aspx?lvl=2&lvlid=62. Accessed March 11, 2020.
8. Falasinnu T, Chaichian Y, Bass MB, et al. The representation of gender and race/ethnic groups in randomized clinical trials of individuals with systemic lupus erythematosus. Curr Rheumatol Rep 2018;20(4):20.
9. Fda, Cder, Fox, Stephanie. Enhancing the Diversity of Clinical Trial Populations-Eligibility Criteria, Enrollment Practices, and Trial Designs Guidance for Industry DRAFT GUIDANCE. Available at: https://www.fda.gov/media/127712/download.
10. Loree JM, Anand S, Dasari A, et al. Disparity of race reporting and representation in clinical trials leading to cancer drug approvals from 2008 to 2018. JAMA Oncol 2019;5(10):e191870.
11. NIH Policy and Guidelines on The Inclusion of Women and Minorities as Subjects in Clinical Research | grants.nih.gov. Available at: https://grants.nih.gov/policy/inclusion/women-and-minorities/guidelines.htm. Accessed March 11, 2020.
12. Chen MS, Lara PN, Dang JHT, et al. Twenty years post-NIH Revitalization Act: Enhancing minority participation in clinical trials (EMPaCT): Laying the groundwork for improving minority clinical trial accrual. Cancer 2014;120:1091–6.
13. Geller SE, Koch AR, Roesch P, et al. The more things change, the more they stay the same: a study to evaluate compliance with inclusion and assessment of women and minorities in randomized controlled trials. Acad Med 2018;93(4):630–5.
14. Fanouriakis A, Kostopoulou M, Alunno A, et al. 2019 update of the EULAR recommendations for the management of systemic lupus erythematosus. Ann Rheum Dis 2019;78(6):736–45.

15. Murphy G, Isenberg DA. New therapies for systemic lupus erythematosus - past imperfect, future tense. Nat Rev Rheumatol 2019;15(7):403–12.
16. Horowitz DL, Furie R. Belimumab is approved by the FDA: what more do we need to know to optimize decision making? Curr Rheumatol Rep 2012;14(4):318–23.
17. Vukelic M, Li Y, Kyttaris VC. Novel treatments in lupus. Front Immunol 2018;9: 2658.
18. Furie R, Khamashta M, Merrill JT, et al. Anifrolumab, an anti–interferon-α receptor monoclonal antibody, in moderate-to-severe systemic lupus erythematosus. Arthritis Rheumatol 2017;69(2):376–86.
19. Furie R, Petri M, Zamani O, et al. A phase III, randomized, placebo-controlled study of belimumab, a monoclonal antibody that inhibits B lymphocyte stimulator, in patients with systemic lupus erythematosus. Arthritis Rheum 2011;63(12): 3918–30.
20. Morand EF, Furie R, Tanaka Y, et al. Trial of anifrolumab in active systemic lupus erythematosus. N Engl J Med 2020;382(3):211–21.
21. Wallace DJ, Furie RA, Tanaka Y, et al. Baricitinib for systemic lupus erythematosus: a double-blind, randomised, placebo-controlled, phase 2 trial. Lancet 2018; 392(10143):222–31.
22. van Vollenhoven RF, Hahn BH, Tsokos GC, et al. Efficacy and safety of ustekinumab, an IL-12 and IL-23 inhibitor, in patients with active systemic lupus erythematosus: results of a multicentre, double-blind, phase 2, randomised, controlled study. Lancet 2018;392(10155):1330–9.
23. Litwic AE, Sriranganathan MK, Edwards CJ. Race and the response to therapies for lupus: how strong is the evidence? Int J Clin Rheumtol 2013;8(4):471–81.
24. Lewis MJ, Jawad AS. The effect of ethnicity and genetic ancestry on the epidemiology, clinical features and outcome of systemic lupus erythematosus. Rheumatology 2016;56(suppl_1):kew399.
25. Yen EY, Singh RR. Brief report: lupus-an unrecognized leading cause of death in young females: a population-based study using nationwide death certificates, 2000-2015. Arthritis Rheumatol 2018;70(8):1251–5.
26. Singh RR, Yen EY. SLE mortality remains disproportionately high, despite improvements over the last decade. Lupus 2018;27(10):1577–81.
27. Yen EY, Shaheen M, Woo JMP, et al. 46-year trends in systemic lupus erythematosus mortality in the United States, 1968 to 2013: a nationwide population-based study. Ann Intern Med 2017;167(11):777–85.
28. Popejoy AB, Fullerton SM. Genomics is failing on diversity. Nature 2016; 538(7624):161–4.
29. Dooley MA, Hogan S, Jennette C, et al. Cyclophosphamide therapy for lupus nephritis: poor renal survival in black Americans. Kidney Int 1997;51(4):1188–95.
30. Influence of race/ethnicity on response to lupus nephritis treatment: the ALMS study. - PubMed - NCBI. Available at: https://www.ncbi.nlm.nih.gov/pubmed/?term=19933596. Accessed March 11, 2020.
31. Appel GB, Contreras G, Dooley MA, et al. Mycophenolate mofetil versus cyclophosphamide for induction treatment of lupus nephritis. J Am Soc Nephrol 2009;20(5):1103–12.
32. Langefeld CD, Ainsworth HC, Cunninghame Graham DS, et al. Transancestral mapping and genetic load in systemic lupus erythematosus. Nat Commun 2017;8:16021.
33. Anjorin A, Lipsky P. Engaging African ancestry participants in SLE clinical trials. Lupus Sci Med 2018;5(1):e000297.

34. Sweeney TE, Khatri P. Generalizable biomarkers in critical care: toward precision medicine. Crit Care Med 2017;45(6):934–9.
35. Vidal AC, Smith JS, Valea F, et al. HPV genotypes and cervical intraepithelial neoplasia in a multiethnic cohort in the southeastern USA. Cancer Causes Control 2014;25(8):1055–62.
36. African American Women Are Less Likely to Benefit From HPV Vaccines for Cervical Cancer Prevention - The ASCO Post. Available at: https://www.ascopost.com/News/8703. Accessed March 11, 2020.
37. Collinson S, Parker B, Mccarthy E, et al. FRI0173 how well do clinical trials represent real world lupus nephritis patients? Ann Rheum Dis 2019;78:760, 1-760.
38. Sheikh SZ, Wanty NI, Stephens J, et al. The state of lupus clinical trials: minority participation needed. J Clin Med 2019;8(8):1245.
39. Mills EJ, Seely D, Rachlis B, et al. Barriers to participation in clinical trials of cancer: a meta-analysis and systematic review of patient-reported factors. Lancet Oncol 2006;7(2):141–8.
40. Ford JG, Howerton MW, Lai GY, et al. Barriers to recruiting underrepresented populations to cancer clinical trials: a systematic review. Cancer 2008;112(2):228–42.
41. Gorelick PB, Harris Y, Burnett B, et al. The recruitment triangle: reasons why African Americans enroll, refuse to enroll, or voluntarily withdraw from a clinical trial: an interim report from the African-American Antiplatelet Stroke Prevention Study (AAASPS). J Natl Med Assoc 1998;90(3):141–5.
42. Battafarano DF, Ditmyer M, Bolster MB, et al. 2015 American College of Rheumatology Workforce Study: supply and demand projections of Adult Rheumatology Workforce, 2015–2030. Arthritis Care Res 2018;70(4):617–26.
43. Alsan M, Garrick O, Graziani G. Does diversity matter for health? Experimental evidence from Oakland. Am Econ Rev 2019;109(12):4071–111.
44. Fouad MN, Acemgil A, Bae S, et al. Patient navigation as a model to increase participation of African Americans in cancer clinical trials. J Oncol Pract 2016;12(6):556–63.
45. Tan MH, Thomas M, MacEachern MP. Using registries to recruit subjects for clinical trials. Contemp Clin Trials 2015;41:31–8.

Designing an Intervention to Improve Management of High-Risk Lupus Patients Through Care Coordination

Allen Anandarajah, MD, MS

KEYWORDS

- Lupus • Health care disparities • Care coordination • High-risk patients • Access

KEY POINTS

- Health care disparities are a major cause for large discrepancies in health outcomes between different populations with systemic lupus erythematosus in the United States.
- A team-based model that incorporates a care coordination strategy in the management of high-risk lupus patients can provide an effective method to overcome the obstacles posed by health care disparities.
- Access, behavioral modification, community outreach programs, depression, and education are key aspects that need to be addressed when designing interventions to improve the quality of care for high-risk lupus patients.

INTRODUCTION

Systemic lupus erythematosus (SLE) or lupus as it is commonly known is a chronic, systemic, autoimmune disease that can affect multiple organ systems. Patients with lupus have a higher morbidity and mortality compared with the general population.[1] Over the past 50 years, advances in diagnostic tests, classification criteria, and therapies have helped decrease the morbidities and mortalities associated with SLE.[2] Large discrepancies in health outcomes, however, still exist between different populations with SLE in the United States. SLE patients from African American and Latinx communities, persons from lower socioeconomic groups, and certain geographic areas are noted to have poorer health outcomes than others with the disease. In recent years, several investigators have set out to identify the underlying causes for these health disparities, resulting in a plethora of articles on this topic. However, there continues to be a paucity of data on practical approaches to overcome these challenges faced by the SLE patients at high risk for poor outcomes. In this article, the author outlines a "roadmap" to consider when designing an intervention to navigate the obstacles posed by health disparities and improve the quality of care for the high-risk SLE population.

Division of Allergy, Immunology & Rheumatology Division, University of Rochester Medical Center, 601 Elmwood Avenue, PO Box 695, Rochester, NY 14642, USA
E-mail address: Allen_Anandarajah@urmc.rochester.edu

Rheum Dis Clin N Am 46 (2020) 723–734
https://doi.org/10.1016/j.rdc.2020.07.012
0889-857X/20/© 2020 Elsevier Inc. All rights reserved.

rheumatic.theclinics.com

DEFINING HIGH-RISK SYSTEMIC LUPUS ERYTHEMATOSUS PATIENTS

A first step in designing a model for management for SLE patients would entail defining the high-risk SLE group. The scientific literature has highlighted the role of race and ethnicity as risk factors for poor outcomes, with African American and Latinx patients known to have higher disease severity, more complications, and a 3- to 4-fold mortality when compared with non-Hispanic whites.[3,4] Although the potential role of genetic, hormonal, and biological factors as causes for poor outcomes among lupus patients needs to be acknowledged, there is mounting evidence to implicate an even bigger effect from environmental triggers, such as socioeconomic status and other social aspects.[5] A list of common determinants for health disparities are shown in **Fig. 1**. Several of these attributes, such as race, ethnicity, socioeconomic status, and geographic area, are interrelated and cannot be easily modified and therefore are not ideal for defining risk groups. Frequent hospitalization and early readmissions are common occurrences among SLE patients with greater disease activity and poor outcomes. These patients who require multiple admissions often have the aforementioned social and environment risk factors. Hospitalizations are also a major contributor to high health care cost, can be measured, and notably can be altered by changes in the health system.[6] Moreover, the number of readmissions is considered an important outcome measure used to assess the quality of care.[7] The author therefore proposes that SLE patients who require multiple hospitalizations be considered a high-risk SLE group.

IDENTIFICATION OF MODIFIABLE RISK FACTORS

The next step is to identify the root causes for health disparities and determine those that are modifiable. Developing programs to address these causes are most likely to result in an overall improvement in health status and subsequently lead to a reduction

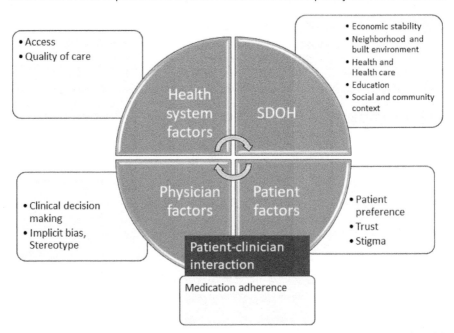

Fig. 1. Factors associated with health care disparities. SDOH, social determinants of health

in hospitalizations and poor outcomes among high-risk SLE patients. Although the distinct measures to be included in the program should be based on the needs of the specific target population, there are common strategies required to lay the foundation when designing a model to improve the quality of care for these patients. The 5 areas to focus are access, behavioral health, community outreach, depression, and education (A–E) (**Fig. 2**). The evidence behind the reasons for focusing on these topics is discussed later.

DESIGNING A SUSTAINABLE INTERVENTION MODEL

An essential final step in designing and maintaining a successful program is to build a financially viable model. Indeed, monetary restrictions and resource limitations are major reasons for the lack of efforts to overcome the common causes for health disparities to date. Restructuring available assets to build a team-based care model offers the best chance to create a sustainable model and minimizes the need for additional resources. Using this team to embrace the goals of care coordination can afford an efficient method to provide high-quality care for high-risk lupus patients.

Care coordination is a patient- and family-centered, team-based activity designed to assess and meet the needs of patients, while helping them navigate effectively and efficiently through the health care system.[8] Care coordination can therefore help bridge the gap between the complex needs of the high-risk lupus patients and the often fragmented health care solutions available to this group. A robust program will be able to help patients overcome gaps in medical, social, behavioral, educational, and financial needs. The goals of the program and abilities of the individual members will determine the components of the care coordination team.

THE AUTHOR'S EXPERIENCE: THE PROJECT TO IMPROVE THE QUALITY OF LOW INCOME, UNDERSERVED, POOR, UNDERPRIVILIDGED SYSTEMIC LUPUS ERYTHEMATOSUS PATIENTS (IQ-LUPUS) MODEL

In 2017, the author started a project to Improve the Quality of Low-income, Underserved, Poor, Underprivileged, SLE patients (IQ-LUPUS). The author identified patients who required 3 or more admissions per year as representing the high-risk

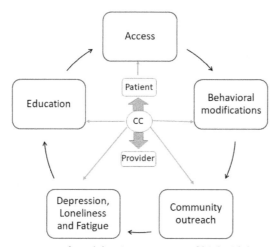

Fig. 2. Essential components of model to improve care of high-risk lupus patients. CC, care coordination

group. The author went on to demonstrate that this group of patients accounted for more admissions, especially 30-day readmissions, and a higher cost compared with the other lupus patients admitted to Strong Memorial Hospital during the same 3-year period (**Table 1**), a high-need, high cost group.

Grant support from the Greater Rochester Health Foundation along with additional support from the University of Rochester Medical Center helped establish a care co-ordination team, the core of which comprised a social worker, a part-time nurse, and 2 physicians. At various stages of the project, the author was also able to get support from pharmacists, data analysts, medical residents and students, community health experts, and community leaders. **Fig. 3** provides the concepts for a proposed care co-ordination model.

An important part of instituting the model was to ensure easy access for the high-risk patients to the coordination team. The team provided all patients and participants with business cards that had direct contact information, with unique phone numbers for the project, to the team members. Patients enrolled in the program were provided clear and concise guidelines on the goals of the project, information on the appropriateness of requests for the team, and the expectations for response time. Team meetings were held every 2 weeks to review problems and advance solutions. In addition, the team established special lupus clinics at a health care center within the city in areas much more accessible to high-risk patients. Work flow in these clinics was modified to address the needs of the SLE patients and maximize the interaction of patients with the care coordination team. In addition, the team developed strategies to address the aforementioned specific risk factors.

ACCESS

The lack of access to health care and failure to receive timely care are key causes of health care disparities. The Institute of Medicine (IOM) committee defines access as the timely use of personal health services to achieve the best possible health outcomes.[9] The reasons for problems with access are complex and can be broadly divided into structural, financial, and personal factors. Structural elements include the geographic location of health services and the availability of health care professionals. Access to primary care physicians and specialists as well as the experience of the physicians and hospitals involved in the care of lupus patients is known to influence outcomes in SLE.[10–12] Financial causes, such as inadequate or lack of insurance coverage, cost of care and of medications, and the monetary status of the patient, can

Table 1
Comparison of high-risk systemic lupus erythematosus patients to other systemic lupus erythematosus patients who required admission to Strong Memorial Hospital between 2014 and 2016

	High-Risk Group	Other SLE Patients
Number of patients	44	158
Total number of admissions	275	192
Total number of 30-d readmissions	105	11
Average number of admissions/patient/y	6.3	1.2
Length of stay (days)	1973	1667
Total cost of all admissions	$6,775,138	$6,417,208
Mean cost per patient	$153,980.41	$40,615.96

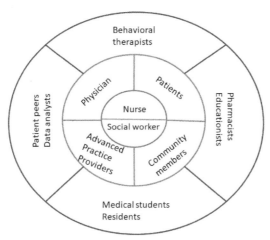

Fig. 3. Proposed care coordination model. Core group: Nurse, social worker, patient, physician, advanced practice providers and community members. Larger group: could include behavioral therapists, pharmacists, educationists, patient peers, data analysts, residents and medical students.

contribute to fewer physician visits and later presentations in disease courses.[13,14] Personal factors comprise the failure to recognize the comorbidities of SLE, childcare and workplace demands, stigma associated with diagnosis, poor physician-patient communication, and a distrust of the health system, all significant hurdles unique to the underserved populations.[15] These patient-related behaviors, perhaps allied to lower educational levels, limited English proficiency, and racism faced by minority communities, result in underutilization of available health care resources. Outlining methods to prevail over the barriers imposed by access-related issues is therefore pivotal in planning a program to improve quality of care to high-risk lupus patients.

A major goal of care coordination is to facilitate timely, appropriate care. Structural problems related to access are often imposing, but careful planning can mitigate these obstacles. Logistical and financial impediments as well as the lack of health care professionals make it almost impossible to secure rheumatology/lupus clinics in all communities with high-risk SLE populations. Linking with community health centers, which are established to serve the needs of underserved inner-city and rural communities, can help optimize health benefits to these populations. Members of the coordinating team can serve as navigators to help patients schedule multiple appointments, including doctor visits, medical tests, and wellness visits and at the same as act as liaisons between the referring providers and lupus experts. The patient navigation system is in fact a community-based service delivery intervention designed to promote access and thereby facilitate timely diagnosis and appropriate treatment of chronic diseases. The coordination team can potentially work with the community center to make available provisions for transportation, translation, and case management services and deliver opportunities for health education and social support as well. The social worker will be able to cater for any additional efforts required to resolve financial and insurance limitations or legal matters that limit access to the specialist. Other than connecting patients to high-quality health organizations and experienced health providers, the care team can also ensure that cultural competency methods are met during clinic visits and accommodate for the complex demands of the high-risk SLE patients. Furthermore, the continuity of care afforded by the coordinating team can boost the provider-patient communication, build trust, and in doing so, improve adherence rates among patients. In summary, the care coordination model, by using the virtues of patient navigation and social work, can attenuate the social, financial, and personal barriers to access faced by high-risk patients with lupus and at the same time foster a great relationship between the community and the health organization.

BEHAVIORAL CHANGES

Unhealthy personal behavior is a major contributor to health disparities and is reported to be directly related to socioeconomic disadvantage.[16] Personal behaviors, such as cigarette smoking, other substance abuse, physical inactivity, obesity, unhealthy food choices, and risky sexual behaviors, are major reasons for premature death and disproportionately impact members of the underserved communities. Similarly, behavior is often a critical consideration in terms of adherence to medication and other therapeutic regimens.[17] Medication adherence rates range from 43% to 75% among patients with lupus but are even lower among members of minority communities.[18] Exploring the basis for these behaviors is beyond the scope of this article. It is however imperative that an effective strategy is devised to reinforce healthy behavioral patterns as part of interventions to optimize care for high-risk lupus patients.

Essential goals of behavioral modification will aim to (1) promote healthy attitudes, such as increased physical activity, healthy diets, smoking cessation, and counseling on drug use; (2) support self-efficacy; and (3) encourage medication adherence. A well-structured care coordination team can help accomplish these goals during interactions at clinic visits and via specially organized sessions. The care coordination team can also use tools from community and national programs, targeted to promote healthy behaviors, to aid patients make necessary lifestyle changes. In addition, self-efficacy programs are powerful means to help patients make lifestyle modifications and embrace a healthier lifestyle. Working closely with the physicians, nurses can develop and oversee formal self-help programs that encourage symptom management, advance communication with physicians, nurture adherence to treatment, and aid efforts to improve physical health components.[19–21] The agenda may also be customized to nurture social support, an important aspect of care for high-risk SLE patients, discussed later.[22,23] Nurses are present in most health care settings, work in close physical proximity to patients, and act as interfaces between patients and physicians. This accessibility of nurses to patients makes them well placed to provide patient education and counseling as well as confer and coordinate adherence care.[19,24] Where possible, enlisting ancillary health care providers, such as pharmacists and behavioral specialists, can further amplify medication adherence rates. Taken together, it is clear that nurse coordinators can be uniquely positioned to help patients develop healthy behaviors and empower them to take care of their own health.

COMMUNITY OUTREACH EFFORTS

The importance of cultural competence as a potential strategy to improve quality is being recognized. Distrust of the health system, lower educational levels, and language barriers are potential reasons for members of minority communities to not participate in preventive health services or not be aware of specific health programs designed for them. As such, projects to serve the minority communities need to be culturally and linguistically appropriate. Health status and disease activity in patients with SLE are also strongly associated with social support.[25] Several studies have highlighted the relationship between inadequate social support and worse physical and mental function, lower self-reported global health, increased psychological distress, and greater disease activity in patients with SLE.[20,26]

Community outreach programs are a great means to serve underserved populations who are less likely to join in the usual channels of health care despite often having a higher disease burden than the general population. A necessary step in the management of high-risk SLE patients is to truly understand the needs of these patients and stimulate their engagement in developing solutions. Outreach programs advance direct engagement with the community and thereby raise the possibility of working in tandem with the local leaders to determine the needs of the at-risk patient population. The coordination team can organize community outreach events in the form of social events, educational sessions, or focus group meetings. The inclusion of family members in these programs can help build a support network for the patients to help them and their loved ones cope with the new diagnosis, clarify treatment options, locate community resources, and garner ongoing support, all of which lead to better health outcomes.[26,27] Such events will also enable conversations, analyze the issues that affect the local community, build trust, and in the process build long-term partnerships, which will help all stakeholders. Focus group meetings are a great way to address specific issues, as the typically smaller settings make it less stress provoking to patients. The close interaction between patients and the coordinating team members at these meetings builds credibility and promotes better patient interaction with the health care systems. In essence, outreach programs can help build a vibrant network of health care providers, patients, friends, relatives, and community members that in turn can raise awareness of the lupus program and bridge the gap between the needs of a community, the availability of a service to help overcome these needs, and the actual use of it.

DEPRESSION, FATIGUE, AND LONELINESS

Depression and other psychological comorbidities are reported to be more prevalent in the lupus populations compared with the general population.[28] African American race and lower socioeconomic status are associated with higher vulnerability for SLE-related depression.[29] Current prevalence levels may be underestimated, because mental problems often tend to masquerade as somatic complaints in those from minority communities. Depression in SLE can be part of neurologic manifestations of lupus, secondary to rashes especially on face, leading to low self-esteem, side effects of medications, or related to emotional and psychological stress of living with a chronic disease. The importance of assessing for and addressing the psychological difficulties faced by patients with SLE is well established.[30]

A robust care coordination model will allow for early screening and diagnosis of depression among the high-risk lupus patients and should be designed to facilitate collaboration with behavioral health providers and primary care physicians to provide the necessary therapy. However, not all patients will need medications or the services of a psychiatrist, and the care coordination team may be able tender multiple solutions. Pain management, overcoming loneliness, and social isolation are important components in the management and prevention of depression. Ensuring availability of social support programs, capacity for self-care, and medication compliance may be sufficient in some patients and complement medical therapies in others. Education of family and friends to understand the symptoms of depression will assist in creating a supportive environment for those facing stigma and loneliness, commonly noted in SLE patients. The social worker can also work with behavioral specialists to expedite crisis intervention and task-centered counseling in those patients who have more severe psychological needs. The ability of a care coordination model to link the typically separate care delivery arrangements for mental and general health care systems permits the holistic approach of care, often sought for by patients.

EDUCATION

The IOM defines health literacy as "the degree to which individuals have the capacity to obtain, process and understand basic information and services needed to make appropriate decisions regarding their health."[31] Low educational levels leads to poor understanding of the disease process and a decrease in the ability to self-manage symptoms and negatively affects communication skills with physicians, all of which are predictive of poor outcomes.[1,20] Hence, the need for planned education activities is an integral part of programs that aim to provide high-quality care to high-risk lupus patients.

Nurses can initiate patient education at clinic visits, at special group therapy sessions, during community events, or as part of self-management classes. Such activities are known to improve patient-provider interactions, enhance patient's understanding of their disease process, and improve adherence rates.[32,33] Educational sessions that are culturally and linguistically appropriate are more likely to be well received and effective. An ideal means to achieve cultural competency is to endorse active engagement of members of the community or patient peers who best understand patient preferences. The process of organizing and providing educational material to patients will also further advance the knowledge of lupus for members of the care coordination team. An often forgotten part of improving care of lupus patients is the need to educate the health care providers. It is important for the lupus team to work with primary care physicians, other specialists, community health workers, and their office staff to lead advocacy efforts to raise awareness of the disease, convey information on early signs and symptoms that will allow for early accurate diagnosis, and facilitate ease of referral to the lupus clinics.

SUCCESSES AND CHALLENGES

The author's program has reaped some early successes. The author was able to demonstrate a reduction in the number of admissions and 30-day readmissions among the high-risk group enrolled in the project (**Fig. 4**A, B) and also noted an improvement in the adherence to outpatient visits among this group (**Fig. 4**C). In addition, patients, community leaders, and community health experts have acknowledged the benefits of the program at various levels.

There are several challenges to implementing a care coordination model for the management of lupus patients. The relatively low prevalence rates, lack of awareness about the complexity of the disease, the limited data on the benefits, and cost-effectiveness of care coordination with regards to high-risk lupus patients can all result in difficulty gaining funds from hospital administrators. In addition, there are several logistical problems that are yet to be clarified. The patient caseloads for coordinators involved in lupus have not been defined. Retrieving and integrating data on quality measures and costs necessary to meet the needs of administrators is often challenging and time consuming for the care coordination team. Devising pilot projects to calculate cost savings through the reduction in admissions and length of stay, determining the revenues generated from increased outpatient visits, and accounting for potential patient and physician satisfaction scores may help secure the necessary finances.

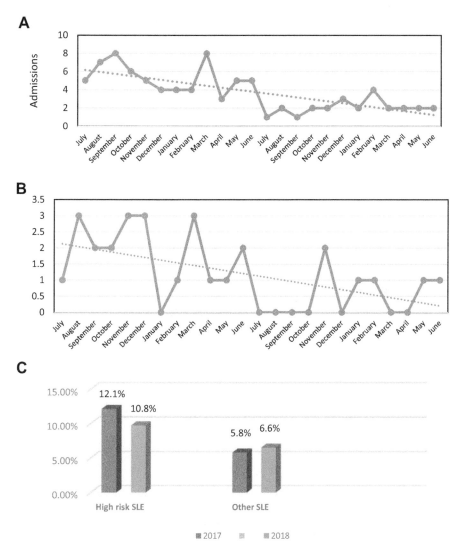

Fig. 4. (*A*) Total number of admissions for the high-risk SLE cohort for the first 2 years of the IQ-LUPUS project. (*B*) Total number of 30-day readmissions for the high-risk cohort over the first 2 years of the IQ-LUPUS project. (*C*) No-show rates to outpatient clinic visits for years 1 and 2 of the IQ-LUPUS project.

SUMMARY

The increasing complexity and fragmentation of the health care system have made care coordination an increasingly valuable tool in the management of patients with chronic illnesses. Lupus is a chronic disease that disproportionately affects young women of color and is associated with worse outcomes among those from lower socioeconomic backgrounds. Thus, it offers a means to comprehend issues related to health care disparities. Management models that incorporate care coordination help facilitate collaboration between the rheumatologists, other specialists, primary care physicians, and patients, which in turn can establish a foundation to a health care delivery system that advances early diagnosis, timely referral, appropriate treatments, and preventive care services for high-risk SLE patients. In addition, well-designed management programs for high-risk lupus populations that incorporate essential elements can empower patients to understand their disease, improve their health-related behaviors, better communicate with physicians, increase adherence with outpatient visits and medication use, and become partners in decision making about their health, all essential components of a patient-centric program.

DISCLOSURE

None to report.

REFERENCES

1. Demas KL, Costenbader KH. Disparities in lupus care and outcomes. Curr Opin Rheumatol 2009;21:102–9.
2. Fiehn C, Hajjar Y, Mueller K, et al. Improved clinical outcome of lupus nephritis during the past decade: importance of early diagnosis and treatment. Ann Rheum Dis 2003;62:435–9.
3. González LA, Toloza SM, Alarcón GS. Impact of race and ethnicity in the course and outcome of systemic lupus erythematosus. Rheum Dis Clin North Am 2014; 40:433–54.
4. Alarcon GS, Friedman AW, Straaton KV, et al. Systemic lupus erythematosus in three ethnic groups: III. A comparison of characteristics early in the natural history of the LUMINA cohort. LUpus in MInority populations: NAture vs. Nurture. Lupus 1999;8:197–209.
5. Alarcon GS, McGwin G Jr, Sanchez ML, et al. Systemic lupus erythematosus in three ethnic groups; XIV. Poverty, wealth and their influence on disease activity. Arthritis Rheum 2004;51:73–7.
6. Anandarajah AP, Luc M, Ritchlin CT. Hospitalization of patients with systemic lupus erythematosus is a major cause of direct and indirect healthcare costs. Lupus 2017;26:756–61.
7. Yazdany J, Marafino BJ, Dean ML, et al. Thirty-day hospital readmissions in systemic lupus erythematosus: predictors and hospital- and state-level variation. Arthritis Rheumatol 2014;66:2828–36.
8. Chapter 2. What is care coordination? Rockville (MD): Agency for Healthcare Research and Quality; 2014. Available at: https://www.ahrq.gov/ncepcr/care/coordination/atlas/chapter2.html.
9. Millman M, editor. Access to health care in America: Institute of Medicine (US) committee on monitoring access to personal health care services. Washington (DC): National Academies Press (US); 1993.
10. Bolster MB, Bass AR, Hausmann JS, et al. 2015 American College of Rheumatology Workforce Study: the role of graduate medical education in adult rheumatology. Arthritis Rheumatol 2018;70:817–25.
11. Ward MM. Association between physician volume and in-hospital mortality in patients with systemic lupus erythematosus. Arthritis Rheum 2005;52:1646–54.
12. Tonner C, Trupin L, Yazdany J, et al. Role of community and individual characteristics in physician visits for persons with systemic lupus erythematosus. Arthritis Care Res 2010;62:888–95.
13. Gillis JZ, Yazdany J, Trupin L, et al. Medicaid and access to care among persons with systemic lupus erythematosus. Arthritis Rheum 2007;57:601–7.

14. Yazdany J, Gillis JZ, Trupin L, et al. Association of socioeconomic and demographic factors with utilization of rheumatology subspecialty care in systemic lupus erythematosus. Arthritis Rheum 2007;57:593–600.
15. Freeman HP. Poverty, culture, and social injustice: determinants of cancer disparities. CA Cancer J Clin 2004;54:72–7.
16. Higgins ST. Behavior change, health and health disparities: an introduction. Prev Med 2014;68:1–4.
17. Marcum ZA, Sevick MA, Handler SM. Medication nonadherence: a diagnosable and treatable medical condition. JAMA 2013;309:2105–6.
18. Mehat P, Atiquzzaman M, Esdaile JM, et al. Medication nonadherence in systemic lupus erythematosus: a systematic review. Arthritis Care Res (Hoboken) 2017;69:1706–13.
19. Eijk-Hustings YV, van Tubergen A, Boström C, et al. EULAR recommendations for the role of the nurse in the management of chronic inflammatory arthritis. Ann Rheum Dis 2012;71:13–9.
20. Karlson EW, Daltroy LH, Lew RA, et al. The relationship of socioeconomic status, race, and modifiable risk factors to outcome in patients with systemic lupus erythematosus. Arthritis Rheum 1997;40:47–56.
21. Williams EM, Dismuke CL, Faith TD, et al. Cost-effectiveness of a peer mentoring intervention to improve disease self-management practices and self-efficacy among African American women with systemic lupus erythematosus. Lupus 2019;28:937–44.
22. Kim SS, Mancuso CA, Huang W-T, et al. Social capital: a novel platform for understanding social determinants of health in systemic lupus erythematosus. Lupus 2015;24:122–9.
23. Drenkard C, Dunlop-Thomas C, Easley K, et al. Benefits of a self-management program in low-income African-American women with systemic lupus erythematosus: results of a pilot study. Lupus 2012;21:1586–93.
24. Verloo H, Chiolero A, Kiszio B, et al. Nurse interventions to improve medication adherence among discharged older adults: a systematic review. Age Ageing 2017;46:747–54.
25. Bae SC, Hashimoto H, Karlson EW, et al. Variable effects of social support by race, economic status, and disease activity in systemic lupus erythematosus. J Rheumatol 2001;28:1245–51.
26. Zheng Y, Ye DQ, Pan HF, et al. Influence of social support on health-related quality of life in patients with systemic lupus erythematosus. Clin Rheumatol 2009;28: 265–9.
27. Phillip CR, Mancera-Cuevas K, Leatherwood C, et al. Implementation and dissemination of an African American popular opinion model to improve lupus awareness: an academic-community partnership. Lupus 2019;28:1441–51.
28. Zhang L, Fu T, Yin R, et al. Prevalence of depression and anxiety in systemic lupus erythematosus: a systematic review and meta-analysis. BMC Psychiatry 2017;17:70.
29. Trupin L, Tonner MC, Yazdany J, et al. The role of neighborhood and individual socioeconomic status in outcomes of systemic lupus erythematosus. J Rheumatol 2008;35:1782–8.
30. Beckerman NL, Auerbach C, Blanco I. Psychosocial dimensions of SLE: implications for the health care team. J Multidiscip Health 2011;4:63–72.
31. Nielsen-Bohlman L, Panzer AM, Kindig DA, Institute of Medicine Committee on Health Literacy. Health literacy: a prescription to end confusion. Washington (DC): National Academic Press; 2004.

32. Hill J, Bird H, Johnson S. Effect of patient education on adherence to drug treatment for rheumatoid arthritis: a randomized controlled trial. Ann Rheum Dis 2001; 60:869–75.
33. Feldman CH1, Bermas BL, Zibit M, et al. Designing an intervention for women with systemic lupus erythematosus from medically underserved areas to improve care: a qualitative study. Lupus 2013;22:52–62.

UNITED STATES POSTAL SERVICE ®
Statement of Ownership, Management, and Circulation
(All Periodicals Publications Except Requester Publications)

1. Publication Title
RHEUMATIC DISEASE CLINICS OF NORTH AMERICA

2. Publication Number
006 - 272

3. Filing Date
9/18/2020

4. Issue Frequency
FEB, MAY, AUG, NOV

5. Number of Issues Published Annually
4

6. Annual Subscription Price
$362.00

7. Complete Mailing Address of Known Office of Publication (Not printer) (Street, city, county, state, and ZIP+4®)
ELSEVIER INC.
230 Park Avenue, Suite 800
New York, NY 10169

Contact Person
Malathi Samayan

Telephone (Include area code)
91-44-4299-4507

8. Complete Mailing Address of Headquarters or General Business Office of Publisher (Not printer)
ELSEVIER INC.
230 Park Avenue, Suite 800
New York, NY 10169

9. Full Names and Complete Mailing Addresses of Publisher, Editor, and Managing Editor (Do not leave blank)

Publisher (Name and complete mailing address)
Dolores Meloni, ELSEVIER INC.
1600 JOHN F KENNEDY BLVD. SUITE 1800
PHILADELPHIA, PA 19103-2899

Editor (Name and complete mailing address)
LAUREN BOYLE, ELSEVIER INC.
1600 JOHN F KENNEDY BLVD. SUITE 1800
PHILADELPHIA, PA 19103-2899

Managing Editor (Name and complete mailing address)
PATRICK MANLEY, ELSEVIER INC.
1600 JOHN F KENNEDY BLVD. SUITE 1800
PHILADELPHIA, PA 19103-2899

10. Owner (Do not leave blank. If the publication is owned by a corporation, give the name and address of the corporation immediately followed by the names and addresses of all stockholders owning or holding 1 percent or more of the total amount of stock. If not owned by a corporation, give the names and addresses of the individual owners. If owned by a partnership or other unincorporated firm, give its name and address as well as those of each individual owner. If the publication is published by a nonprofit organization, give its name and address.)

Full Name	Complete Mailing Address
WHOLLY OWNED SUBSIDIARY OF REED/ELSEVIER, US HOLDINGS	1600 JOHN F KENNEDY BLVD. SUITE 1800 PHILADELPHIA, PA 19103-2899

11. Known Bondholders, Mortgagees, and Other Security Holders Owning or Holding 1 Percent or More of Total Amount of Bonds, Mortgages, or Other Securities. If none, check box ▶ ☐ None

Full Name	Complete Mailing Address
N/A	

12. Tax Status (For completion by nonprofit organizations authorized to mail at nonprofit rates) (Check one)
The purpose, function, and nonprofit status of this organization and the exempt status for federal income tax purposes:
☒ Has Not Changed During Preceding 12 Months
☐ Has Changed During Preceding 12 Months (Publisher must submit explanation of change with this statement)

PS Form **3526**, July 2014 [Page 1 of 4 (see instructions page 4)] PSN: 7530-01-000-9931 PRIVACY NOTICE: See our privacy policy on www.usps.com.

---

13. Publication Title
RHEUMATIC DISEASE CLINICS OF NORTH AMERICA

14. Issue Date for Circulation Data Below
MAY 2020

15. Extent and Nature of Circulation

			Average No. Copies Each Issue During Preceding 12 Months	No. Copies of Single Issue Published Nearest to Filing Date
a.	Total Number of Copies (Net press run)		179	165
b. Paid Circulation (By Mail and Outside the Mail)	(1)	Mailed Outside-County Paid Subscriptions Stated on PS Form 3541 (include paid distribution above nominal rate, advertiser's proof copies, and exchange copies)	85	79
	(2)	Mailed In-County Paid Subscriptions Stated on PS Form 3541 (include paid distribution above nominal rate, advertiser's proof copies, and exchange copies)	0	0
	(3)	Paid Distribution Outside the Mails Including Sales Through Dealers and Carriers, Street Vendors, Counter Sales, and Other Paid Distribution Outside USPS®	56	51
	(4)	Paid Distribution by Other Classes of Mail Through the USPS (e.g. First-Class Mail®)	0	0
c.	Total Paid Distribution (Sum of 15b (1), (2), (3), and (4)) ▶		141	130
d. Free or Nominal Rate Distribution (By Mail and Outside the Mail)	(1)	Free or Nominal Rate Outside-County Copies included on PS Form 3541	24	21
	(2)	Free or Nominal Rate In-County Copies included on PS Form 3541	0	0
	(3)	Free or Nominal Rate Copies Mailed at Other Classes Through the USPS (e.g. First-Class Mail)	0	0
	(4)	Free or Nominal Rate Distribution Outside the Mail (Carriers or other means)	24	21
e.	Total Free or Nominal Rate Distribution (Sum of 15d (1), (2), (3) and (4)) ▶		24	21
f.	Total Distribution (Sum of 15c and 15e) ▶		165	151
g.	Copies not Distributed (See Instructions to Publishers #4 (page 3)) ▶		14	14
h.	Total (Sum of 15f and g) ▶		179	165
i.	Percent Paid (15c divided by 15f times 100) ▶		85.45%	86.09%

* If you are claiming electronic copies, go to line 16 on page 3. If you are not claiming electronic copies, skip to line 17 on page 3.

16. Electronic Copy Circulation

		Average No. Copies Each Issue During Preceding 12 Months	No. Copies of Single Issue Published Nearest to Filing Date
a.	Paid Electronic Copies ▶		
b.	Total Paid Print Copies (Line 15c) + Paid Electronic Copies (Line 16a) ▶		
c.	Total Print Distribution (Line 15f) + Paid Electronic Copies (Line 16a) ▶		
d.	Percent Paid (Both Print & Electronic Copies) (16b divided by 16c × 100) ▶		

☒ I certify that 50% of all my distributed copies (electronic and print) are paid above a nominal price.

17. Publication of Statement of Ownership
☒ If the publication is a general publication, publication of this statement is required. Will be printed
in the NOVEMBER 2020 issue of this publication.
☐ Publication not required.

18. Signature and Title of Editor, Publisher, Business Manager, or Owner

Malathi Samayan - Distribution Controller

Malathi Samayan

Date 9/18/2020

I certify that all information furnished on this form is true and complete. I understand that anyone who furnishes false or misleading information on this form or who omits material or information requested on the form may be subject to criminal sanctions (including fines and imprisonment) and/or civil sanctions (including civil penalties).

PS Form **3526**, July 2014 (Page 3 of 4) PRIVACY NOTICE: See our privacy policy on www.usps.com

Moving?

Make sure your subscription moves with you!

To notify us of your new address, find your **Clinics Account Number** (located on your mailing label above your name), and contact customer service at:

Email: journalscustomerservice-usa@elsevier.com

800-654-2452 (subscribers in the U.S. & Canada)
314-447-8871 (subscribers outside of the U.S. & Canada)

Fax number: 314-447-8029

Elsevier Health Sciences Division
Subscription Customer Service
3251 Riverport Lane
Maryland Heights, MO 63043

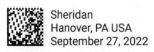